M000228028

Milady's Standard Esthetics

FUNDAMENTALS

Step-by-Step Procedures

10th Edition

Milady's Standard Esthetics

FUNDAMENTALS

Joel Gerson

Step-by-Step Procedures

Contributors:
Janet D'Angelo
Sallie Deitz
Shelley Lotz

Editorial Contributor:
Letha Barnes

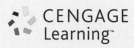
CENGAGE
Learning™

Australia • Brazil • Japan • Korea • Mexico • Singapore • Spain • United Kingdom • United States

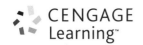
CENGAGE
Learning™

Milady's Standard Esthetics: Fundamentals Step-by-Step Procedures, Tenth Edition
Joel Gerson, Janet D'Angelo, Sallie Deitz, Shelley Lotz, and Letha Barnes

President, Milady: Dawn Gerrain

Publisher: Erin O'Connor

Acquisitions Editor: Martine Edwards

Editorial Assistant: Beth Nutting-Edwards

Director of Beauty Industry Relations: Sandra Bruce

Senior Marketing Manager: Gerard McAvey

Marketing Specialist: Erica Conley

Production Director: Wendy Troeger

Senior Content Project Manager: Nina Tucciarelli

Art Director: Joy Kocsis

© 2010 Delmar, Cengage Learning

ALL RIGHTS RESERVED. No part of this work covered by the copyright herein may be reproduced, transmitted, stored, or used in any form or by any means graphic, electronic, or mechanical, including but not limited to photocopying, recording, scanning, digitizing, taping, Web distribution, information networks, or information storage and retrieval systems, except as permitted under Section 107 or 108 of the 1976 United States Copyright Act, without the prior written permission of the publisher.

For product information and technology assistance, contact us at
Professional & Career Group Customer Support, 1-800-648-7450

For permission to use material from this text or product,
submit all requests online at **www.cengage.com/permissions**
Further permissions questions can be e-mailed to
permissionrequest@cengage.com

Library of Congress Control Number: 2007941007

ISBN-13: 978-1-4390-5925-8

ISBN-10: 1-4390-5925-X

Milady
5 Maxwell Drive
Clifton Park, NY 12065-2919
USA

Cengage Learning products are represented in Canada by Nelson Education, Ltd.

For your lifelong learning solutions, visit **www.milady.cengage.com**
Visit our corporate website at **www.cengage.com**

Notice to the Reader
Publisher does not warrant or guarantee any of the products described herein or perform any independent analysis in connection with any of the product information contained herein. Publisher does not assume, and expressly disclaims, any obligation to obtain and include information other than that provided to it by the manufacturer. The reader is expressly warned to consider and adopt all safety precautions that might be indicated by the activities described herein and to avoid all potential hazards. By following the instructions contained herein, the reader willingly assumes all risks in connection with such instructions. The publisher makes no representations or warranties of any kind, including but not limited to, the warranties of fitness for particular purpose or merchantability, nor are any such representations implied with respect to the material set forth herein, and the publisher takes no responsibility with respect to such material. The publisher shall not be liable for any special, consequential, or exemplary damages resulting, in whole or part, from the readers' use of, or reliance upon, this material.

Printed in the United States of America
1 2 3 4 5 QWD 13 12 11 10 09

Procedures List

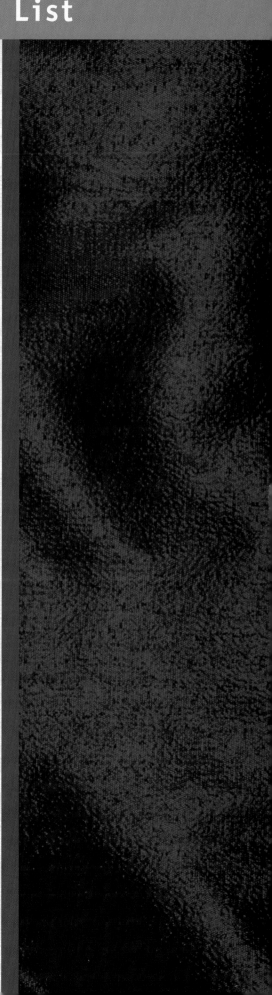

Procedures List

How to Use This Book

Congratulations on purchasing this step-by-step procedures book, a companion to your *Milady's Standard Esthetics: Fundamentals*, 10th Edition, textbook. You can use this book in conjunction with your textbook, or on its own to brush up on key procedures. Each step is clearly explained and is accompanied throughout by full-color photos.

PERFORMANCE RUBRICS

At the end of each procedure, you'll find a list of rubrics, or ways to note and comment on your performance for each of the key tasks. Rubrics are used in education for organizing and interpreting data gathered from observations of student performance. Rubrics are specifically developed scoring documents used to differentiate between levels of development in a specific skill performance or behavior. You can use rubrics to evaluate yourself, other estheticians, and other students. As an instructor, you can use rubrics to evaluate your own students.

WHAT'S ON THE DVD?

To assist you in really learning each and every step, we've noted which procedures can be found on the companion DVD set, *Milady's Standard Esthetics: Fundamentals*. If you already own these DVDs, or know that your school owns them, we encourage you to watch the procedure in video to strengthen your understanding of that particular procedure.

OTHER COMPANION PRODUCTS

Other products in this same product line may be of interest to you, the practicing or future esthetician:

Milady's Standard Esthetics: Fundamentals, 10th Edition
Joel Gerson
ISBN-13: 9781428318922
ISBN-10: 1428318925
©2009

Milady's Standard Esthetics: Fundamentals, DVD Series
Milady
ISBN-13: 9781435402812
ISBN-10: 1435402812
©2009

Milady's Standard Esthetics: Fundamentals, Student Workbook
Milady
ISBN-13: 9781428318946
ISBN-10: 1428318941
©2009

*Milady's Standard Esthetics: Fundamentals Online Licensing
   Preparation*, Slimline
Milady
ISBN-13: 9781428319073
ISBN-10: 1428319077
©2009

Milady's Standard Esthetics: Fundamentals, Exam Review
Milady
ISBN-13: 9781428318953
ISBN-10: 142831895X
©2009

Milady's Standard Esthetics: Fundamentals, Student CD ROM
Milady
ISBN-13: 9781428318977
ISBN-10: 1428318976
©2009

Milady's Standard Esthetics: Fundamentals, Spanish Version
Milady
ISBN-13: 9781428319028
ISBN-10: 1428319026
©2009

Milady's Standard Esthetics: Fundamentals, Exam Review Spanish Version
Milady
ISBN-13: 9781428318960
ISBN-10: 1428318968
©2009

Milady's Standard Esthetics: Fundamentals, Student Workbook, Spanish Version
Milady
ISBN-13: 9781562538378
ISBN-10: 1428318941
©2009

Milady's Standard Esthetics: Advanced
Milady
ISBN-13: 9781428319752
ISBN-10: 1428319751
©2010

For more products serving practicing and future estheticians, please visit www.milady.cengage.com

Photo Credits:

Procedure 4–2-1: Larry Hamill Photography, Columbus, Ohio

Procedures 13–1 and 13–2: Paul Castle Photography, Troy, NY

Procedure 14–8: Paul Castle Photography, Troy, NY

Procedure 15–1: Paul Castle Photography, Troy, NY

Procedure 17–6: Paul Castle Photography, Troy, NY

All other photos by Rob Werfel Photography, Ashland, Oregon.

Step-by-Step Procedures

IMPLEMENTS AND MATERIALS

Most tools and implements can be disinfected. These include scissors, tweezers, plastic spatulas, and other nonporous implements.

SUPPLIES

- gloves
- disinfectant
- disinfectant container
- water
- soap
- paper towels
- safety goggles
- implements

Any item that is used on a client must be disinfected or discarded after each use. Items that cannot be disinfected, such as sponges or cotton swabs, must be discarded. Electrodes, tweezers, and other nonporous tools must be sterilized or disinfected.

All implements should be thoroughly cleaned before soaking to avoid contaminating the disinfecting solution. Creams, oils, and makeup lessen the effectiveness of the solution. Always disinfect your tools or other implements according to the guidelines listed for EPA wet disinfectants. This means complete immersion for the required amount of time. The following are guidelines for specific salon materials.

Preparation

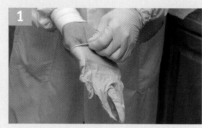

Put on gloves, goggles, or safety glasses. *(Figure P4–1-1)*

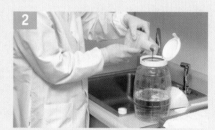

Always add disinfectant to water. *(Figure P4–1-2)*

1. Put on gloves, goggles, or safety glasses (Figure P4-1-1).

2. Mix disinfectant according to manufacturer's directions, always adding disinfectant to the water in the disinfectant container so no disinfectant can splash up or out of the container. (Figure P4-1-2).

Procedure

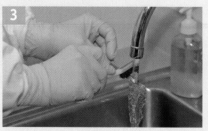

Pre-clean to remove all visible debris and residue from tools and implements. *(Figure P4-1-3)*

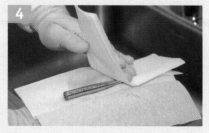

Rinse items thoroughly and pat dry with a clean towel. *(Figure P4-1-4)*

3. Pre-clean to remove hair, filings and debris, and other such loose matter by scrubbing implements with soap and water (Figure P4-1-3).

4. Rinse items thoroughly and pat dry with a clean towel (Figure P4-1-4).

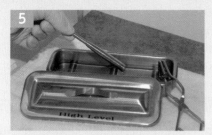

Completely immerse implements or
tools for the required amount of time.
(Figure P4–1-5)

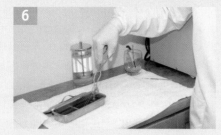

Remove implements with tongs, basket,
or gloves. *(Figure P4–1-6)*

5 Using gloves or tongs, completely immerse implements or
tools and leave for the required
amount of time, per manufacturer's instructions (Figure P4–1-5).

6 Remove implements with clean
tongs, basket, or gloves so as
not to contaminate the disinfectant. Rinse thoroughly and dry
(Figure P4–1-6).

Clean-Up

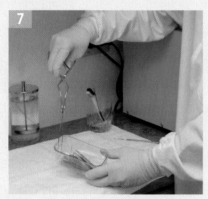

Place disinfected implements in a
clean, closed, dry, disinfected container.
(Figure P4–1-7)

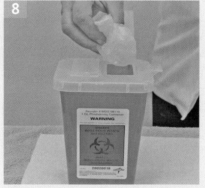

Clean up the workstation, including
glove disposal and other disinfectant
measures. *(Figure P4–1-8)*

7 Place disinfected implements
in a clean, closed, dry, disinfected container (such as a
plastic container with a lid)
(Figure P4–1-7).

8 Clean up the workstation,
including glove disposal and
other disinfectant measures
(Figure P4–1-8).

Rubrics are used in education for organizing and interpreting data gathered from observations of student performance. It is a clearly developed scoring document used to differentiate between levels of development in a specific skill performance or behavior. Rubrics are provided in this supplement for use as either a self-assessment tool to aid the student in behavior development or as an educator assessment tool to determine competence. Space is provided to record steps needed for further growth and improvement.

Rate performance according to the following scale:

1   **Development Opportunity:** There is little or no evidence of competency; Assistance is needed; Performance includes multiple errors.

2   **Fundamental:** There is beginning evidence of competency; Task is completed alone; Performance includes few errors.

3   **Competent:** There is detailed and consistent evidence of competency; Task is completed alone; Performance includes rare errors.

4   **Strength:** There is detailed evidence of highly creative, inventive, mature presence of competency.

Space is provided for comments to assist you in improving your performance and achieving a higher rating.

PERFORMANCE ASSESSED	1	2	3	4	IMPROVEMENT PLAN
Preparation					
1. Put on gloves, goggles, or safety glasses.					
2. Mixed disinfectant according to manufacturer's directions.					
3. Added disinfectant to water.					
Procedure					
1. Pre-cleaned implements to remove hair, filings, debris by scrubbing with soap and water.					
2. Rinsed items thoroughly.					
3. Patted items dry with clean towel.					
4. Using gloves or tongs, completely immersed implements or tools.					
5. Immersed implements for required amount of time.					
6. Removed implements with clean tongs, basket, or gloves.					
7. Rinsed implements thoroughly.					
8. Dried implements thoroughly.					
Clean-Up and Sanitation					
1. Placed disinfected implements in a clean, closed, dry, disinfected container.					
2. Cleaned up workstation.					
3. Properly disposed of gloves and other disposables.					

SUPPLIES

- cotton
- swabs
- sponges
- gauze
- brushes
- spatulas
- tweezers
- comedo extractors
- electrodes
- wax strips
- gloves

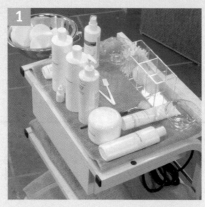

Lay out implements and materials before beginning a service. *(Figure P4–2-1)*

An **aseptic procedure** is the process of properly handling sterilized and disinfected equipment and supplies so that they do not become contaminated by microorganisms before they are used on a client. The following is a good example of an aseptic procedure.

1 Set up for the service. Before beginning any treatment, wash your hands using proper sanitizing methods. Lay out on a clean towel all implements that you will use during the treatment (Figure P4–2-1), such as cotton, swabs, sponges, and so forth. To prevent airborne contact, cover with another clean towel until you are ready to start the treatment. By pre-arranging these utensils, you will be less likely to need to open a container to get more supplies. This not only prevents cross-contamination but is also more efficient. Once you have begun a treatment, never open any package or container or touch a product without a spatula or tongs. Touching any object with gloved hands that have touched the client will contaminate that object. Any object touched during treatment must be discarded, disinfected, or autoclaved.

Procedure

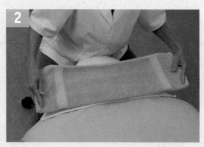

Use clean towels, sheets, headband or plastic cap, and gown for each client. *(Figure P4–2-2)*

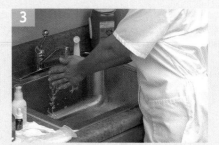

Wash and sanitize your hands after touching a client's hair. *(Figure P4–2-3)*

2 Use clean towels, sheets, headband or plastic cap, and gown for each client (Figure P4–2-2).

3 Wash and sanitize your hands after touching a client's hair (Figure P4–2-3).

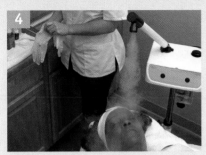

Gloves should be worn for safety and hygiene. *(Figure P4–2-4)*

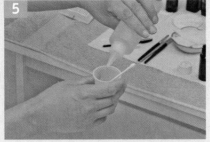

Remove products before the treatment and place them in small disposable cups. *(Figure P4–2-5)*

4 Put on gloves at the beginning of every treatment, and wear them throughout the treatment (Figure P4–2-4). This is especially important during and after extraction, waxing, or electrolysis.

5 Remove creams and products from containers using pumps, squeeze bottles with dispenser caps, or disinfected spatulas. It is best to remove products before the treatment and place them in small disposable cups (Figure P4–2-5). This way you will not have to touch bottles or jars with soiled gloved hands. Spatulas should be disinfected or discarded after each use.

Clean-Up

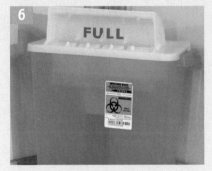

Dispose of lancets and other sharp implements in a sharps box. *(Figure P4–2-6)*

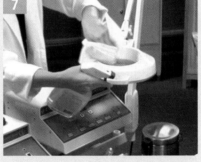

Wipe down all surfaces touched during treatment with a disinfectant before your next client. *(Figure P4–2-7)*

6 After completing the treatment, place linens in a covered laundry receptacle. Throw away disposable items in a closed trash container. Place sharps in a sharps box (Figure P4–2-6). Disinfect or sterilize all items to be reused. Discard any unused product that has been removed from its container.

7 Wipe down all surfaces touched during treatment with a disinfectant before the next client is seated (Figure P4–2-7).

Rubrics are used in education for organizing and interpreting data gathered from observations of student performance. It is a clearly developed scoring document used to differentiate between levels of development in a specific skill performance or behavior. Rubrics are provided in this supplement for use as either a self-assessment tool to aid the student in behavior development or as an educator assessment tool to determine competence. Space is provided to record steps needed for further growth and improvement.

Rate performance according to the following scale:

1 **Development Opportunity:** There is little or no evidence of competency; Assistance is needed; Performance includes multiple errors.

2 **Fundamental:** There is beginning evidence of competency; Task is completed alone; Performance includes few errors.

3 **Competent:** There is detailed and consistent evidence of competency; Task is completed alone; Performance includes rare errors.

4 **Strength:** There is detailed evidence of highly creative, inventive, mature presence of competency.

Space is provided for comments to assist you in improving your performance and achieving a higher rating.

PERFORMANCE ASSESSED	1	2	3	4	IMPROVEMENT PLAN
Preparation					
1. Gathered equipment, supplies, disposables, and products.					
2. Completed proper hand washing.					
3. Laid out all implements and supplies needed for service.					
4. Covered implements with another clean towel until beginning service.					
5. Never touched a product without using a sterile spatula or tongs.					
Procedure					
1. Used clean linens.					
2. Washed and sanitized hands after touching client.					
3. Put on gloves at beginning of treatment.					
4. Wore gloves throughout treatment.					
5. Removed products and placed in small disposable cups prior to treatment.					
Clean-Up and Sanitation					
1. Placed linens in covered receptacle.					
2. Discarded all disposable items properly.					
3. Placed sharps in a sharps box.					
4. Disinfected all items to be reused.					
5. Discarded any unused products removed from containers.					
6. Wiped down all surfaces touched during treatment with disinfectant.					

4-2

SUPPLIES
- paper towels
- soap
- nail brush
- warm water

Procedure

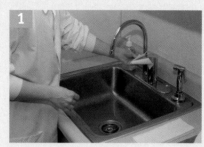

Turn faucet on with a clean, dry paper towel. *(Figure P4–3-1)*

1 Use a paper towel to turn faucet on, if it is not automatic (Figure P4-3-1).

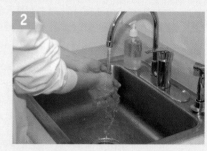

Dampen hands with warm water. *(Figure P4–3-2)*

2 Dampen hands with warm water (Figure P4-3-2).

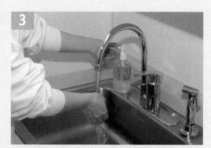

Apply soap and massage hands thoroughly, including nails and fingers. *(Figure P4–3-3)*

3 Apply soap and massage hands thoroughly, including nails and fingers (Figure P4-3-3).

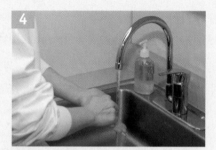

Lather with soap and scrub hands for 20–30 seconds. *(Figure P4–3-4)*

4 Lather with soap and scrub hands thoroughly for 20 to 30 seconds (Figure P4-3-4).

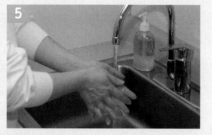

Rinse hands with warm water. *(Figure P4–3-5)*

5 Rinse hands with warm water (Figure P4-3-5).

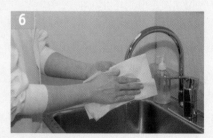

Dry with paper towel. *(Figure P4-3-6)*

6 Dry hands with paper towel (Figure P4-3-6).

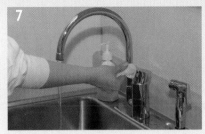

7 Turn faucet off using an additional clean paper towel (Figure P4–3-7).

Turn faucet off with additional clean paper towel. *(Figure P4-3-7)*

? **Did You Know**

As of January 2008, OSHA required all health workers to use nitrile gloves as a response to the growing allergic reactions to other materials such as latex. **Nitrile gloves** are made from synthetic rubbers, known as *acrylonitrile* and *butadiene,* and are resistant to tears, punctures, chemicals, and solvents.

Clean-Up

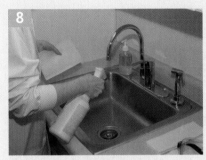

8 Disinfect sink after each service (Figure P4–3-8).

Disinfect sink after each service. *(Figure P4-3-8)*

CAUTION!

All gloves are to be removed by turning them inside out and pulling them off. Think dirty to dirty, and clean to clean. After removing gloves, dispose of them in the appropriately marked (biohazard) trash can. This prevents the transfer of microorganisms and accidental contamination.

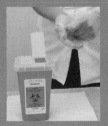

Pull top of glove inside out from the outside with opposite gloved hand.

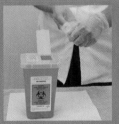

Pull glove completely off inside out with opposite gloved hand.

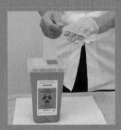

With free hand, pull off remaining glove, touching only the inside.

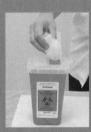

Dispose off gloves in an appropriate biohazard container.

Rubrics are used in education for organizing and interpreting data gathered from observations of student performance. It is a clearly developed scoring document used to differentiate between levels of development in a specific skill performance or behavior. Rubrics are provided in this supplement for use as either a self-assessment tool to aid the student in behavior development or as an educator assessment tool to determine competence. Space is provided to record steps needed for further growth and improvement.

Rate performance according to the following scale:

1 **Development Opportunity:** There is little or no evidence of competency; Assistance is needed; Performance includes multiple errors.

2 **Fundamental:** There is beginning evidence of competency; Task is completed alone; Performance includes few errors.

3 **Competent:** There is detailed and consistent evidence of competency; Task is completed alone; Performance includes rare errors.

4 **Strength:** There is detailed evidence of highly creative, inventive, mature presence of competency.

Space is provided for comments to assist you in improving your performance and achieving a higher rating.

PERFORMANCE ASSESSED	1	2	3	4	IMPROVEMENT PLAN
Preparation					
1. Gathered supplies.					
Procedure					
1. Used paper towel to turn on faucet if not automatic.					
2. Dampened hands with warm water.					
3. Applied soap and massaged hands thoroughly.					
4. Lathered with soap and scrubbed hands for 20 to 30 seconds.					
5. Rinsed hands with warm water.					
6. Dried hands with paper towel.					
7. Turned off faucet using a clean paper towel.					
Clean-Up and Sanitation					
1. Disinfected sink.					

4-3

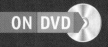
SUPPLIES

(Use this list for all cleansing procedures.)

- disinfectant/sanitizer
- hand sanitizer/antibacterial soap
- covered trash container
- bowl
- spatula
- hand towels
- headband
- clean linens
- bolster

DISPOSABLES

- gloves
- cotton pads
- cotton rounds
- cotton swabs
- plastic bag
- paper towels
- tissues

PRODUCTS

- eye makeup remover or cleanser
- facial cleanser
- toner
- moisturizer

Preparation

1 Prepare the bed and room.

2 Set out the supplies and products on a sanitary maintenance area (SMA).

3 Prepare the client and cover the hair.

Procedure

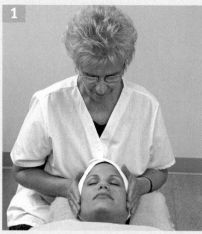

Look at the client's skin before starting the treatment. *(Figure P11–1-1)*

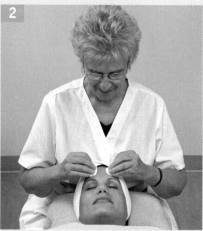

Cleanse the skin. *(Figure P11–1-2)*

1 *Look* briefly at your client's skin with your naked eye or a magnifying light (Figure P11-1-1). You cannot do an accurate analysis if your client is wearing makeup.

2 *Cleanse* the skin (a client's normal state of dryness or oiliness may not be as visible after cleansing) (Figure P11-1-2).

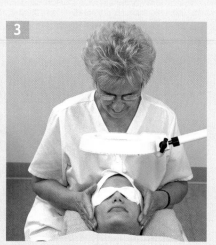

Use the magnifying lamp for a skin analysis. *(Figure P11-1-3)*

3 Use a *magnifying* light to examine the skin more thoroughly (Figure P11-1-3). *Cover the eyes* with eye pads. (In addition to the magnifying light, a Wood's lamp can be used here.)

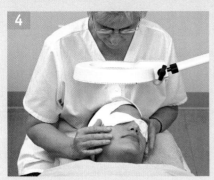

Feel the texture of the skin.
(Figure P11–1-4)

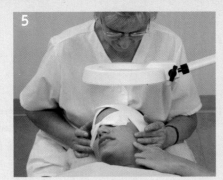

Conduct a brief consultation.
(Figure P11–1-5)

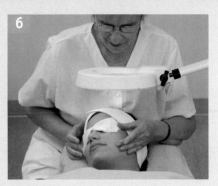

Ask questions during the analysis.
(Figure P11–1-6)

4 *Look* closely at the client's skin type, the conditions present and the appearance; also *touch* the skin with the fingertips to feel its texture (Figure P11–1-4).

5 *Listen*: Conduct a brief *consultation* while continuing to analyze with the magnifying light (Figure P11–1-5). (A Wood's lamp can be used here to see conditions not visible with the naked eye.)

6 *Ask questions* relating to the skin's appearance and the client's personal health. Discuss what you see with the client; also recommend products and a home-care routine (Figure P11–1-6).

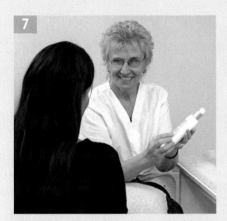

Choosing products for treatment and home care. *(Figure P11–1-7)*

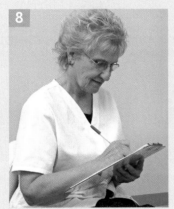

Note information on the client chart. *(Figure P11–1-8)*

FYI

The four components of skin analysis are *look, feel, ask,* and *listen.*

11–1

7 *Choose products* for treatment and home care (Figure P11–1-7).

8 *Record* the information on the client chart at the appropriate time—usually after the treatment is completed (Figure P11–1-8).

Clean-Up

9 Follow the aseptic procedure to avoid contamination. You will follow the same clean-up and sanitation steps as presented in the basic facial procedure (see Procedure 14–4).

Rubrics are used in education for organizing and interpreting data gathered from observations of student performance. It is a clearly developed scoring document used to differentiate between levels of development in a specific skill performance or behavior. Rubrics are provided in this supplement for use as either a self-assessment tool to aid the student in behavior development or as an educator assessment tool to determine competence. Space is provided to record steps needed for further growth and improvement.

Rate performance according to the following scale:

1 **Development Opportunity:** There is little or no evidence of competency; Assistance is needed; Performance includes multiple errors.

2 **Fundamental:** There is beginning evidence of competency; Task is completed alone; Performance includes few errors.

3 **Competent:** There is detailed and consistent evidence of competency; Task is completed alone; Performance includes rare errors.

4 **Strength:** There is detailed evidence of highly creative, inventive, mature presence of competency.

Space is provided for comments to assist you in improving your performance and achieving a higher rating.

PERFORMANCE ASSESSED	1	2	3	4	IMPROVEMENT PLAN
Preparation					
1. Gathered equipment, supplies, disposables, and products.					
2. Prepared bed and room.					
3. Set out supplies and products on sanitary maintenance area.					
4. Sanitized own hands.					
5. Prepared client and covered hair.					
Procedure					
1. Observed client's skin with naked eye.					
2. Cleansed client's skin.					
3. Covered client's eyes with eye pads.					
4. Examined client's skin with magnifying light.					
5. Examined client's skin texture through touch.					
6. Asked questions relating to skin appearance and client's health.					
7. Discussed observations with client.					
8. Recommended home-care routine.					
9. Recommended home-care products.					
10. Recorded information on client chart after treatment.					

PERFORMANCE ASSESSED	1	2	3	4	IMPROVEMENT PLAN
Clean-Up and Sanitation					
1. Discarded all disposable supplies and materials.					
2. Closed product containers, cleaned, and stored properly.					
3. Placed used towels and other linens in covered hamper.					
4. Disinfected workstation and facial table.					
5. Washed own hands with soap and warm water.					

11-1

SUPPLIES

- roll of cotton
- bowl
- water
- disinfectant
- sanitary maintenance area
- covered container or zip-lock plastic bag for storage

Preparation of Cotton Pads and Compresses

If prepackaged 4" × 4" esthetic wipes or sponges are not available, cotton pads can be made from a roll of cotton. You can prepare all cotton cleansing pads, eye pads, and the cotton compress pads that are used in a facial before the treatment begins. In a busy salon, the esthetician should check the appointment book at the beginning of each workday to see how many appointments are booked for that day. To save time, enough pads and compresses can then be made for the entire day if they are kept sanitary. Store pads and compresses in a covered container.

Remove enough pads from the container before each treatment, and place them in a plastic, steel, or glass bowl that is kept within easy reach during the facial treatment. For each client, you may need a minimum of one pair of eye pads, one cotton compress mask, and four to six cleansing pads. The pads and compresses that are not used on the day they are made can be stored safely in an airtight, covered container, or placed in a zip-lock plastic bag and refrigerated for use the next day.

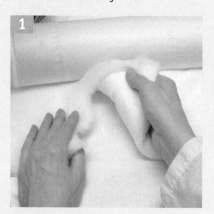

Divide cotton. *(Figure P13–1-1)*

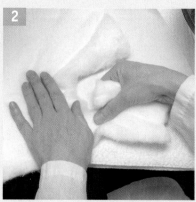

Tear cotton. *(Figure P13–1-2)*

1 Divide a roll of cotton into strips approximately 4" wide. This is about the width of the average hand. Tear the cotton (do not cut) so that the edges are frayed and the cleansing pads are less lumpy when the edges are folded under (Figure P13–1-1).

2 To make cleansing pads, hold one of the cotton strips in one hand and pull downward with the hand until the cotton tears, making a cotton square approximately 4" wide by 5" long. Four to six of these pieces will be needed for each facial treatment (Figure P13–1-2).

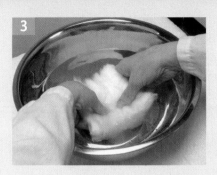

Submerge in water. *(Figure P13–1-3)*

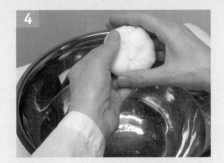

Tuck edges. *(Figure P13–1-4)*

3　Submerge the cotton in water while supporting the pad with your fingers (Figure P13–1-3).

4　Tuck the edges of the cotton under while turning it in your hands (Figure P13–1-4). Place the round pad in the palm of your hand, placing the other palm over the pad. Squeeze out excess water from the pad.

Rubrics are used in education for organizing and interpreting data gathered from observations of student performance. It is a clearly developed scoring document used to differentiate between levels of development in a specific skill performance or behavior. Rubrics are provided in this supplement for use as either a self-assessment tool to aid the student in behavior development or as an educator assessment tool to determine competence. Space is provided to record steps needed for further growth and improvement.

Rate performance according to the following scale:

1 **Development Opportunity:** There is little or no evidence of competency; Assistance is needed; Performance includes multiple errors.

2 **Fundamental:** There is beginning evidence of competency; Task is completed alone; Performance includes few errors.

3 **Competent:** There is detailed and consistent evidence of competency; Task is completed alone; Performance includes rare errors.

4 **Strength:** There is detailed evidence of highly creative, inventive, mature presence of competency.

Space is provided for comments to assist you in improving your performance and achieving a higher rating.

PERFORMANCE ASSESSED	1	2	3	4	IMPROVEMENT PLAN
Preparation					
1. Gathered equipment, supplies, disposables, and products.					
2. Prepared workstation.					
3. Washed hands thoroughly.					
Procedure					
1. Divided roll of cotton into 4" wide strips.					
2. Tore cotton so edges were frayed.					
3. Smoothed cotton to remove lumps.					
4. Tore cotton strip into sections approximately 4" wide by 5" long.					
5. Submerged cotton pad in water while supporting pad with fingers.					
6. Tucked edges of cotton under while turning it in hands.					
7. Placed round pad in palm of hand.					
8. Placed other palm over pad.					
9. Squeezed out excess water from pad.					
Clean-Up and Sanitation					
1. Closed cotton container and stored appropriately.					
2. Disinfected workstation.					
3. Washed own hands with soap and warm water.					

13-1

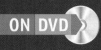
SUPPLIES

- roll of cotton
- bowl
- water
- disinfectant
- sanitary maintenance area
- covered container or zip-lock plastic bag for storage

Eye pads can be made from either 4" × 4" cotton squares, prepackaged round cotton pads, or pieces of cotton. There are two types of eye pads: round and butterfly. Both styles of eye pads are correct, and the choice of which to use is up to the esthetician. The pads should be large enough to cover the entire eye area, but not so large that they interfere with product application or treatment. The advantage of the butterfly pad over the round pad is that it will not fall off of the eyes as easily. Round eye pads are made following the same procedure as for round cleansing pads, but the cotton piece should measure about 2½" × 2½".

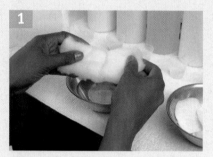

Dip cotton into water. *(Figure P13-2-1)*

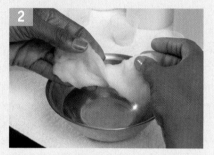

Twist. *(Figure P13-2-2)*

1 Dip a piece of cotton measuring approximately 2" × 6" into the water (Figure P13-2-1).

2 Twist the cotton in the center with a one-half turn (Figure P13-2-2).

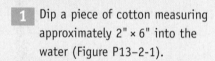

3 Fold the pad in half and squeeze out the excess water (Figure P13-2-3).

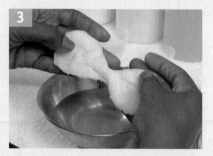

Butterfly pads. *(Figure P13-2-3)*

Optional: Take a square 4" × 4" pad, unfold lengthwise, and twist it in the middle.

Clean-Up

Follow aseptic procedures after the service.

Rubrics are used in education for organizing and interpreting data gathered from observations of student performance. It is a clearly developed scoring document used to differentiate between levels of development in a specific skill performance or behavior. Rubrics are provided in this supplement for use as either a self-assessment tool to aid the student in behavior development or as an educator assessment tool to determine competence. Space is provided to record steps needed for further growth and improvement.

Rate performance according to the following scale:

1 **Development Opportunity:** There is little or no evidence of competency; Assistance is needed; Performance includes multiple errors.

2 **Fundamental:** There is beginning evidence of competency; Task is completed alone; Performance includes few errors.

3 **Competent:** There is detailed and consistent evidence of competency; Task is completed alone; Performance includes rare errors.

4 **Strength:** There is detailed evidence of highly creative, inventive, mature presence of competency.

Space is provided for comments to assist you in improving your performance and achieving a higher rating.

PERFORMANCE ASSESSED	1	2	3	4	IMPROVEMENT PLAN
Preparation					
1. Gathered equipment, supplies, disposables, and products.					
2. Prepared workstation.					
3. Washed hands thoroughly.					
Procedure					
1. Tore a 6" wide strip from the roll of cotton.					
2. Tore 6" strip lengthwise into 2" wide strips.					
3. Tore cotton so edges were frayed.					
4. Smoothed cotton to remove lumps.					
5. Submerged cotton strip in water while supporting pad with fingers.					
6. Twisted cotton strip in center with a one-half turn.					
7. Folded strip in half.					
8. Squeezed out excess water from pad.					
Clean-Up and Sanitation					
1. Closed cotton container and stored appropriately.					
2. Disinfected workstation.					
3. Washed own hands with soap and warm water.					

13–2

SUPPLIES

(Use this list for all cleansing procedures.)

- disinfectant/sanitizer
- hand sanitizer/antibacterial soap
- covered trash container
- bowl
- spatula
- hand towels
- headband
- clean linens
- bolster

DISPOSABLES

- gloves
- cotton pads
- cotton rounds
- cotton swabs
- plastic bag
- paper towels
- tissues

PRODUCTS

- eye makeup remover or cleanser
- facial cleanser

Preparation

1. Prepare the bed and room.

2. Set out supplies and products on an SMA.

3. Prepare the client and cover the hair.

Procedure

Eye Makeup Removal

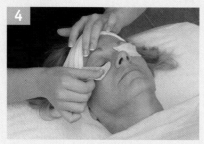

Cleanse the eyelid and lashes. *(Figure P14–1-1)*

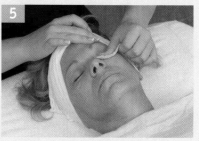

Apply the product to the eyelid with downward strokes. *(Figure P14–1-2)*

4. Bring the left hand over and lift the right eyebrow with the middle and ring fingers. With the middle and ring fingers of the right hand, apply the product to the eyelid with downward strokes (Figure P14–1-1). Use downward movements with the cleansing pad to cleanse the eyelid and lashes. Gently rinse with cotton pads.

5. Move the middle and ring fingers of the right hand over to the left side of the face and lift the left eyebrow. With the middle fingers of the left hand, apply the product to the left lid with downward strokes (Figure P14–1-2). If the client is wearing contacts, do not remove the eye makeup.

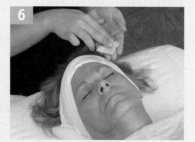

Repeat cleansing. *(Figure P14–1-3)*

6. Repeat this step as necessary to remove eye makeup. While cleansing the eyes, rotate the pad to provide a clean, unused surface (Figure P14-1-3).

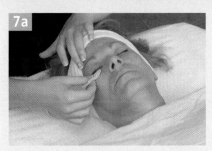

Remove mascara under the eyes. *(Figure P14–1-4)*

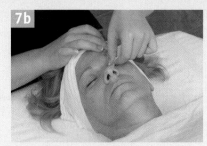

Make a complete circular pattern. *(Figure P14–1-5)*

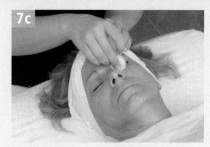

Rinse with water. *(Figure P14–1-6)*

7a Place the edge of the pad under the lower lashes at the outside corner of the eyes, and slide the pad toward the inner corner of the eyes. The mascara will gradually work loose and can be wiped clean. Be especially gentle when cleansing the eyes because the skin around the eyes is very sensitive and can become irritated (Figure P14–1-4). Remove any makeup underneath the eyes. Always be gentle around the eyes; never rub or stretch the skin, as it is very delicate and thin.

7b Use the cotton pad or a cotton swab to wipe inward under the eye toward the nose and then outward on the top of the eyelid (Figure P14–1-5). Making a complete circular pattern.

7c Rinse the eye area with plain water to remove the eye makeup remover (Figure P14–1-6). Make sure the remover is rinsed off thoroughly.

Lipstick Removal

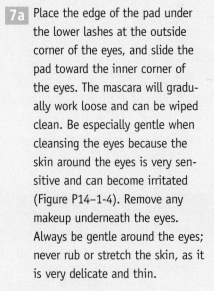

Remove lipstick. *(Figure P14–1-7)*

2 With the index and middle finger (either the left or right side) of one hand, hold on next to the outside edge of the lips to keep the skin tight so it does not move around; then remove with even strokes from the corners of the lips toward the center.

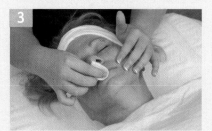

Repeat on other side. *(Figure P14–1-8)*

1 To remove lipstick, apply eye makeup remover or a cleanser to a damp cotton pad or tissue and gently remove the client's lipstick (Figure P14–1-7).

3 Repeat the procedure on the other side until the lips are clean (Figure P14–1-8).

Clean-Up and Sanitation

Follow the clean-up procedure described in the basic facial procedure (see Procedure 14–4).

PROCEDURE 14–1: EYE MAKEUP AND LIPSTICK REMOVAL

Rubrics are used in education for organizing and interpreting data gathered from observations of student performance. It is a clearly developed scoring document used to differentiate between levels of development in a specific skill performance or behavior. Rubrics are provided in this supplement for use as either a self-assessment tool to aid the student in behavior development or as an educator assessment tool to determine competence. Space is provided to record steps needed for further growth and improvement.

Rate performance according to the following scale:

1 **Development Opportunity:** There is little or no evidence of competency; Assistance is needed; Performance includes multiple errors.

2 **Fundamental:** There is beginning evidence of competency; Task is completed alone; Performance includes few errors.

3 **Competent:** There is detailed and consistent evidence of competency; Task is completed alone; Performance includes rare errors.

4 **Strength:** There is detailed evidence of highly creative, inventive, mature presence of competency.

Space is provided for comments to assist you in improving your performance and achieving a higher rating.

PERFORMANCE ASSESSED	1	2	3	4	IMPROVEMENT PLAN
Preparation					
1. Gathered equipment, supplies, disposables, and products.					
2. Prepared the bed.					
3. Prepared the room.					
4. Set out supplies and products.					
5. Cleansed own hands.					
6. Prepared client and covered hair.					
Eye Makeup Removal Procedure					
1. Using left hand, lifted right eyebrow with the middle and ring fingers.					
2. Using middle and ring fingers of right hand, applied cleanser to eyelid with downward strokes.					
3. Cleansed eyelid and lashes with cleansing pad applied in downward movements.					
4. Using right hand, lifted left eyebrow with the middle and ring fingers.					
5. Using middle and ring fingers of left hand, applied cleanser to the eyelid with downward strokes.					
6. Cleansed eyelid and lashes with cleansing pad applied in downward movements.					
7. Repeated cleansing steps as necessary.					
8. Rotated pad while cleansing to provide a clean, unused surface.					

PERFORMANCE ASSESSED	1	2	3	4	IMPROVEMENT PLAN
9. Placed the edge of the pad under lower lashes at the outside corner of the eyes.					
10. Slid the pad toward the inner corner of the eyes.					
11. Removed any makeup under the eyes.					
12. Did not rub or stretch the skin.					
13. Using cotton pad or swab, completed the circular pattern.					
14. Rinsed the eye area with plain water to remove product thoroughly.					
Lipstick Removal Procedure					
1. Applied cleanser to damp cotton pad or tissue.					
2. With index and middle finger of one hand, held outside edge of the lips taut.					
3. Removed lipstick with even strokes from corners of lips toward center.					
4. Repeated procedure on the opposite side of lips.					
5. Continued until lips were clean.					
Clean-Up and Sanitation					
1. Discarded all disposable supplies and materials.					
2. Closed product containers, cleaned and stored properly.					
3. Placed used towels and other linens in covered hamper.					
4. Disinfected workstation and facial table.					
5. Washed own hands with soap and warm water.					

14-1

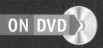

SUPPLIES

- disinfectant/sanitizer
- hand sanitizer/antibacterial soap
- covered trash container
- bowl
- spatula
- hand towels
- headband
- clean linens
- bolster

DISPOSABLES

- gloves
- cotton pads
- cotton rounds
- cotton swabs
- plastic bag
- paper towels
- tissues

PRODUCTS

- eye makeup remover or cleanser
- facial cleanser
- toner
- moisturizer

The following method of application is used when applying cleansers, massage creams, treatment creams, and protective products. Most product removal requires rinsing each area at least three times. If possible, use both hands at the same time. The hands must be clean before touching the client's face.

Preparation

1. Prepare the bed and room.

2. Set out supplies and products on an SMA.

3. Prepare the client and cover the hair.

Procedure

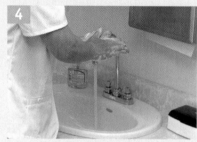

Sanitize hands. *(Figure P14-2-1)*

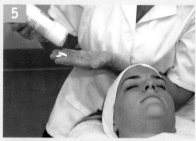

Apply product to fingers. *(Figure P14-2-2)*

4. Cleanse and sanitize the hands before touching the client's face (Figure P14-2-1). Apply warm towels. After checking the temperature, apply one towel to the décolleté and one to the face.

5. Apply approximately one-half teaspoon of the product to the fingers or palms of the hand. Water-soluble cleansing lotion is preferred when cleansing the face because it can be easily removed with moistened cotton pads or sponges (Figure P14-2-2).

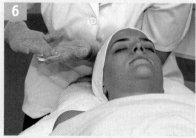

Use circular motion to distribute product. *(Figure P14-2-3)*

6. Use circular motions to distribute the product onto the fingertips. You are now ready to apply the product to the client's décolleté, neck, and face (Figure P14-2-3).

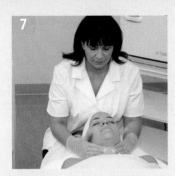

Apply product on neck. *(Figure P14–2-4)*

7 Start applying the product by placing both hands, palms down, on the neck. Slide hands back toward the ears until the pads of the fingers rest at a point directly beneath the ear-lobes (Figure P14–2-4). While applying the product, do not lift your hands from the client's face until you are finished.

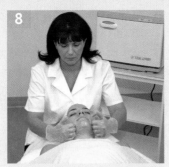

Slide fingers along jawline. *(Figure P14–2-5)*

8 Reverse the hand, with the back of the fingers now resting on the skin, and slide the fingers along the jawline to the chin (Figure P14-2-5).

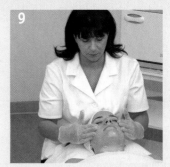

Slide fingers over cheeks. *(Figure P14–2-6)*

9 Reverse the hands again and slide the fingers back over the cheeks until the pads of the fingers come to rest directly in front of the ears (Figure P14-2-6).

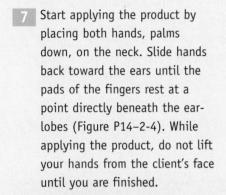

Slide fingers over cheekbones to the nose. *(Figure P14-2-7)*

10 Reverse the hands again, and slide the fingers forward over the cheekbones to the nose (Figure P14-2-7).

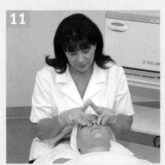

Make small, circular motions on the flare of the nostrils. *(Figure P14–2-8)*

11 With the pads of the middle fingers, make small, circular motions on the top of the nose and on each side of the nose (Figure P14-2-8). Avoid pushing the product into the nose.

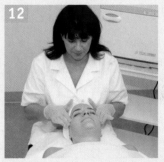

Slide fingers to the forehead and out toward the temple. *(Figure P14–2-9)*

12 Slide the fingers up to the fore-head and outward toward the temples, pausing with a slight pressure on the temples. Slide fingers across the forehead using circles or long strokes from side to side (Figure P14-2-9).

Clean-Up and Sanitation

Follow the clean-up procedure described in the basic facial procedure (see Procedure 14–4).

14-2

PROCEDURE 14–2: APPLYING CLEANSING PRODUCT

Rubrics are used in education for organizing and interpreting data gathered from observations of student performance. It is a clearly developed scoring document used to differentiate between levels of development in a specific skill performance or behavior. Rubrics are provided in this supplement for use as either a self-assessment tool to aid the student in behavior development or as an educator assessment tool to determine competence. Space is provided to record steps needed for further growth and improvement.

Rate performance according to the following scale:

1 **Development Opportunity:** There is little or no evidence of competency; Assistance is needed; Performance includes multiple errors.

2 **Fundamental:** There is beginning evidence of competency; Task is completed alone; Performance includes few errors.

3 **Competent:** There is detailed and consistent evidence of competency; Task is completed alone; Performance includes rare errors.

4 **Strength:** There is detailed evidence of highly creative, inventive, mature presence of competency.

Space is provided for comments to assist you in improving your performance and achieving a higher rating.

PERFORMANCE ASSESSED	1	2	3	4	IMPROVEMENT PLAN
Preparation					
1. Gathered equipment, supplies, disposables, and products.					
2. Prepared the bed and room.					
3. Set out supplies and products.					
4. Helped client prepare for the service.					
5. Properly covered client's hair.					
Procedure					
1. Cleansed own hands.					
2. Applied warm towel to décolleté.					
3. Applied warm towel to face.					
4. Applied cleanser to fingertips.					
5. Used circular motion to distribute product.					
6. Applied product on neck.					
7. Slid hands back toward ears until pads of fingers rested beneath earlobes.					
8. Slid backs of fingers along jawline to chin.					
9. Slid pads of fingers back over cheeks to rest directly in front of ears.					
10. Slid backs of fingers forward over cheekbones to the nose.					
11. Using pads of middle fingers, made small circular movements on top and sides of nose.					

| --- | --- | --- | --- | --- | --- |
12. Slid fingers to the forehead and outward to temples; paused with slight pressure on temples.					
13. Slid fingers across forehead using circles or long strokes from side to side.					
Completion					
1. Washed own hands.					
2. Informed client service was complete and gave instructions for dressing.					
3. Discussed home-care products and regimen.					
Clean-Up and Sanitation					
1. Discarded all disposable supplies and materials.					
2. Closed product containers, cleaned, and stored properly.					
3. Placed used towels and other linens in covered hamper.					
4. Disinfected workstation and facial table.					
5. Washed own hands with soap and warm water.					

14–2

Rinse each area at least three times. Some estheticians prefer to use wet cotton pads or disposable facial sponges when removing product. Others prefer to use towels. Both methods are correct and equally professional, and many estheticians use both methods. For example, an esthetician who usually uses the sponges will use cotton pads when working on acne skin. Even when using sponges, an esthetician may need some cotton during the treatment for eye pads or extracting blackheads.

Movements are generally done in an upward and outward direction from the center to the edges of the face. Under the eyes, it is usually inward to avoid tugging on the eye area.

Procedure

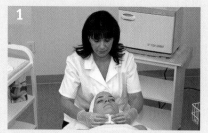

Cleanse the neck. *(Figure P14-3-1)*

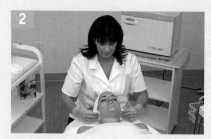

Slide pad along the jawline. *(Figure P14-3-2)*

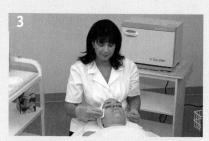

Use upward movements to cleanse the cheeks. *(Figure P14-3-3)*

1 Starting at the décolleté, cleanse sideways and up to the neck. Cleanse the neck using upward strokes. To keep the pad from slipping from the hand, pinch the edge of the pad between the thumb and upper part of the forefinger. It is important that most of the surface of the pad remain in contact with the skin. Do not exert pressure on the Adam's apple (Figure P14-3-1).

2 Place the pad directly under the chin and slide the pad along the jawline, stopping directly under the ear. Repeat the movement on the other side of the face. Alternate back and forth three times on each side of the face, or do the movement concurrently by using both hands at the same time (Figure P14-3-2).

3 Starting at the jawline, use upward movements to cleanse the cheek (Figure P14-3-3).

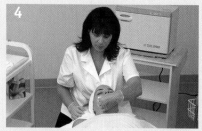

Cross over the chin to the other cheek. *(Figure P14-3-4)*

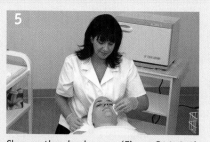

Cleanse the cheek area. *(Figure P14-3-5)*

4 Continuing the upward movement, cross over the chin to the other cheek (Figure P14-3-4).

5 Continue the cleansing movement with approximately six strokes on each cheek (Figure P14-3-5).

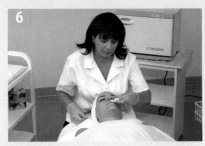

Cleanse underneath the nose. *(Figure P14–3-6)*

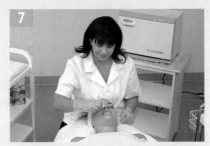

Cleanse the sides of the nose. *(Figure P14–3-7)*

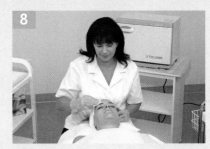

Cleanse the forehead. *(Figure P14–3-8)*

6 Cleanse the area directly underneath the nose by using downward and sideways strokes. Start at the center and work outward toward the corners of the mouth. Alternate the movements back and forth three times on each side of the face (Figure P14–3-6).

7 Starting on the bridge of the nose, cleanse the sides of the nose and the area directly next to it. Use light, outward movements (Figure P14–3-7).

8 Place the pads flat on the center of the forehead, and slide them outward to the temples. Apply a slight pressure on the pressure points of the temples. Repeat the movement three times on each side of the forehead (Figure P14–3-8).

Clean-Up and Sanitation

Follow the clean-up procedure described in the basic facial procedure (see Procedure 14–4).

Rubrics are used in education for organizing and interpreting data gathered from observations of student performance. It is a clearly developed scoring document used to differentiate between levels of development in a specific skill performance or behavior. Rubrics are provided in this supplement for use as either a self-assessment tool to aid the student in behavior development or as an educator assessment tool to determine competence. Space is provided to record steps needed for further growth and improvement.

Rate performance according to the following scale:

1 **Development Opportunity:** There is little or no evidence of competency; Assistance is needed; Performance includes multiple errors.

2 **Fundamental:** There is beginning evidence of competency; Task is completed alone; Performance includes few errors.

3 **Competent:** There is detailed and consistent evidence of competency; Task is completed alone; Performance includes rare errors.

4 **Strength:** There is detailed evidence of highly creative, inventive, mature presence of competency.

Space is provided for comments to assist you in improving your performance and achieving a higher rating.

PERFORMANCE ASSESSED	1	2	3	4	IMPROVEMENT PLAN
Preparation					
1. Gathered equipment, supplies, disposables, and products.					
2. Prepared the bed and room.					
3. Set out supplies and products.					
4. Helped client prepare for the service.					
5. Properly covered client's hair.					
Procedure					
1. Cleansed own hands.					
2. Applied cleanser according to Procedure 14–2.					
3. Starting at décolleté, cleansed sideways and up to the neck.					
4. Cleansed neck using upward strokes.					
5. To prevent slipping, pinched edge of pad between thumb and forefinger.					
6. Did not exert pressure on Adam's apple.					
7. Placed pad directly under chin and slid along jawline, stopping under ear.					
8. Repeated movement on opposite side of face.					
9. Alternated back and forth three times on each side of face, *or* performed movement concurrently with both hands.					
10. Started at jawline and cleansed cheeks using upward movements.					

PERFORMANCE ASSESSED	1	2	3	4	IMPROVEMENT PLAN
11. Continued upward movement, crossed over chin to other cheek.					
12. Continued cleansing with approximately six strokes on each cheek.					
13. Cleansed area beneath nose, using downward and sideways strokes.					
14. Started at center and worked outward toward corner of mouth.					
15. Alternated movements back and forth three times on each side of face.					
16. Started at bridge of nose and cleansed sides of nose and area directly next to it.					
17. Placed pads flat on center of forehead and slid outward to temple.					
18. Applied slight pressure at temples.					
19. Repeated movement three times on each side of forehead.					
Completion					
1. Washed own hands.					
2. Informed client service was complete and gave instructions for dressing.					
3. Discussed home-care products and regimen.					
Clean-Up and Sanitation					
1. Discarded all disposable supplies and materials.					
2. Closed product containers, cleaned, and stored properly.					
3. Placed used towels and other linens in covered hamper.					
4. Disinfected workstation and facial table.					
5. Washed own hands with soap and warm water.					

14–3

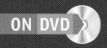
EQUIPMENT
- facial equipment (towel warmer, steamer, magnifying light)

SUPPLIES
- disinfectant/sanitizer
- hand sanitizer/antibacterial soap
- covered trash container
- bowls
- spatulas
- fan and mask brush
- implements
- distilled water
- sharps container
- hand towels
- clean linens
- blanket
- headband
- client gown or wrap
- bolster
- client charts

DISPOSABLES
- cotton pads
- cotton rounds
- cotton swabs
- paper towels
- tissue
- gloves/finger cots
- baggies

PRODUCTS
- cleanser
- exfoliant
- masks
- massage lotion
- toner
- moisturizer
- sunscreen
- optional: serums, eye cream, lip balm, extraction supplies

Now that you have practiced the preliminary steps and cleansing, it is time to put it all together in a complete facial. The steps for performing a basic facial treatment are listed here. Some procedures may vary, however, so be guided by your instructor.

Preparation

1 Set up the room.

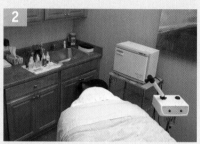

Prepare the treatment room. *(Figure P14–4-1)*

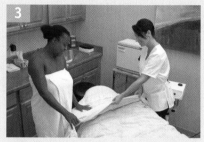

Help the client prepare for the service. *(Figure P14–4-2)*

2 Prepare the bed, equipment, and workstation (Figure P14–4-1).

3 Help the client prepare for the service (Figure P14–4-2).

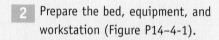

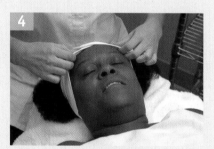

Put on the headband. *(Figure P14-4-3)*

4 Put on the headband (Figure P14–4-3).

Procedure

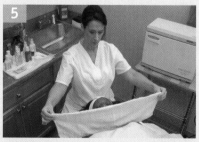

Apply warm towels. *(Figure P14–4-4)*

5 **Cleanse your hands and apply warm towels.** After checking the temperature, apply one towel to the décolleté and one to the face (Figure P14–4-4).

Optional: Remove eye makeup and lipstick. If your client has no makeup, skip this part and proceed to step 5. Remember to ask about contact lenses before putting product on the eyes. If the client is wearing contacts, do not remove the eye makeup.

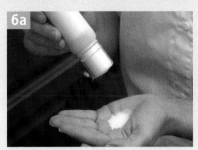
Apply cleanser to fingertips. *(Figure P14–4-5)*

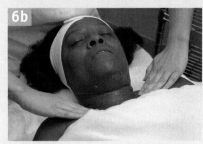
Start at the neck or décolleté. *(Figure P14–4-6)*

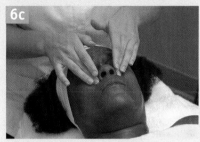
Make small, circular movements with fingertips. *(Figure P14–4-7)*

6 **Cleanse.**

a. Remove about one-half teaspoon of cleanser from the container (with a sanitized spatula if it is not a squirt-top or pump-type lid). Place it in the palm and then apply a small amount to your fingertips (Figure P14–4-5). This conserves the amount of product you use.

b. Starting at the neck or décolleté and with a sweeping movement, use both hands to spread the cleanser upward and outward on the chin, jaws, cheeks, and temples (Figure P14–4-6). Spread the cleanser down the nose and along its sides and bridge.

c. Make small, circular movements with the fingertips around the nostrils and sides of the nose (Figure P14–4-7). Continue with upward-sweeping movements between the brows and across the forehead to the temples.

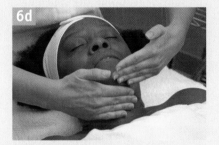
Apply more cleanser with long strokes. *(Figure P14–4-8)*

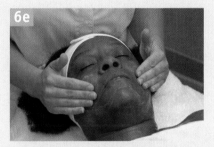
Continue moving up toward the forehead. *(Figure P14–4-9)*

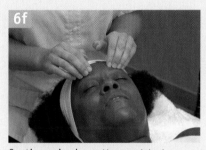
Continue circular pattern out to temples. *(Figure P14–4-10)*

d. Apply more cleanser to the neck and chest with long, even strokes (Figure P14–4-8). Cleanse the area in small, circular motions from the center of the chest and neck toward the outside, moving upward. Try to use both hands at the same time on each side when applying or removing product.

e. Visually divide the face into left and right halves from the center. Continue moving upward with circular motions on the face from the chin and cheeks, and up toward the forehead using both hands, one on each side (Figure P14–4-9).

f. Starting at the center of the forehead, continue with the circular pattern out to the temples (Figure P14–4-10). Move the fingertips lightly in a circle around the eyes to the temples and then back to the center of the forehead. Lift your hands slowly off of the face when you finish cleansing.

Note Remember that procedures vary. In cleansing, the instructor may have you use mainly long strokes, rather than circles.

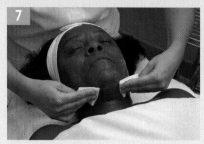

Remove the cleanser. *(Figure P14–4-11)*

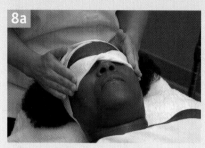

Place eye pads on client. *(Figure P14–4-12)*

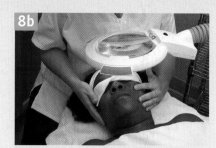

Use the magnifying light to determine skin type and condition. *(Figure P14–4-13)*

7 **Remove the cleanser.** Using moist cotton pads or disposable facial sponges, start at the neck or forehead and follow the contours of the face. Move up or down the face in a consistent pattern, depending on where you start according to the instructor's procedures (Figure P14–4-11). Remove all the cleanser from one area of the face before proceeding to the next. (Under the nostrils, use downward strokes when applying or removing products to avoid pushing product up the nose. This is uncomfortable and will make the client tense.) Blot your hands on a clean towel, and touch the face with dry fingertips to make sure there is no residue left.

8 **Analyze the skin.** Cover the client's eyes with eye pads (Figure P14-4-12). Position the magnifying light where you want it before starting the facial, so that you can swing it over easily to line up over the face (Figure P14-4-13). Note the skin type and condition, and feel the texture of the skin.

Optional: Cleanse the face again. Some treatment protocols do not include this second cleansing. Be guided by your instructor.

Optional: If exfoliation is part of the service, it could be done at this time before steaming. If eyebrow arching is needed, it could be done either at this time or following the steam and extractions to avoid irritation from the steam. Be careful what you apply to waxed areas.

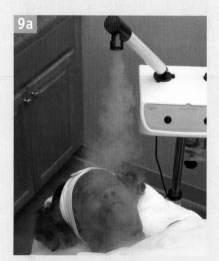

Steam the face. *(Figure P14–4-14)*

9 Steam the face (Figure P14–4-14).

a. Preheat the steamer before you need it. Turn it on, wait for it to start steaming, and then turn on the ozone button if applicable.

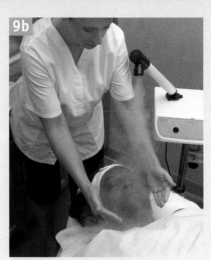

9b

Check that steam reaches both sides of face. *(Figure P14–4-15)*

b. Check to make sure the steamer is not too close to the client (approximately 18 inches away) and that it is steaming the face evenly. If you hold your hands close to the sides of the client's face, you can feel if the steam is reaching both sides of the face (Figure P14–4-15). Steam for approximately 5 to 10 minutes.

c. Turn off the steamer immediately after use. (Review the section on steamers in Chapter 16 for steamer cautions.)

If using towels, remember to test them for the correct temperature. Ask the client if she is comfortable with the temperature. Towels are left on for approximately 2 minutes. Steam or warm towels should be used carefully on couperose skin.

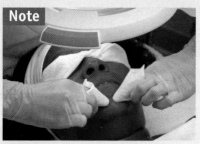

Performing extractions. *(Figure P14–4-16)*

Note Extractions are done immediately after the steam, while the skin is still warm (Figure P14–4-16). Refer to the extractions section of this chapter to incorporate this step into your basic facial procedure if it is applicable to your facility.

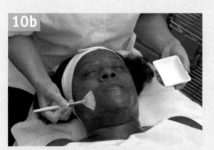

10b

Apply massage cream. *(Figure P14–4-17)*

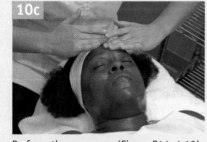

10c

Perform the massage. *(Figure P14–4-18)*

10 **Massage the face.** Use the facial manipulations described in Chapter 15.

a. Select a water-soluble massage cream or product appropriate to the client's skin type.

b. Use the same procedure as you did for product application to apply the massage cream to the face, neck, shoulders, and chest. Apply the warmed product in long, slow strokes with a brush, moving in a set pattern (Figure P14–4-17).

c. Perform the massage as directed (Figure P14–4-18).

10d

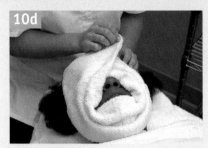

Remove massage cream. *(Figure P14–4-19)*

d. Remove the massage cream. Use warm towels or cleansing pads and follow the same procedure as for removing other products or cleanser (Figure P14–4-19).

11 Apply a treatment mask.

a. Choose a mask formulated for the client's skin condition. Remove the mask from its container, and place it in the palm or a small mixing cup. (Use a clean spatula, if necessary, to avoid contamination.) Warming the mask is recommended.

11b

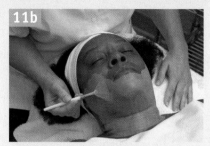

Applying a mask. *(Figure P14–4-20)*

b. Apply the mask with fingers or a brush, usually starting at the neck. Use long, slow strokes from the center of the face, moving outward to the sides (Figure P14–4-20).

11c

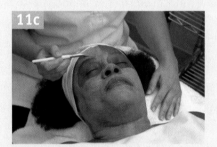

Apply mask from the center outward. *(Figure P14–4-21)*

c. Proceed to the jawline and apply the mask on the face from the center outward (Figure P14-4-21). Avoid the eye area unless the mask is appropriate for that area.

11d

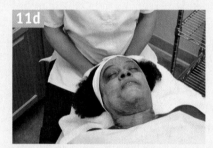

Leave mask on for 7–10 minutes. *(Figure P14–4-22)*

d. Allow the mask to remain on the face for approximately 7 to 10 minutes (Figure P14-4-22).

11e

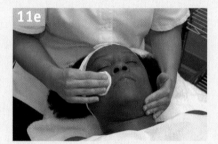

Remove the mask. *(Figure P14–4-23)*

e. Remove the mask with wet cotton pads, sponges, or towels (Figure P14-4-23).

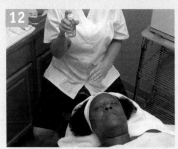

Apply toner. *(Figure P14–4-24)*

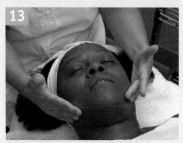

Apply moisturizer and sunscreen.
(Figure P14–4-25)

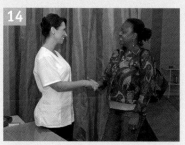

Discuss home-care products and regime.
(Figure P14–4-26)

12 Apply the toner product appropriate for the skin type (Figure P14–4-24).

Note Serums as well as eye and lip creams are optional for application before the final moisturizer.

13 Apply a moisturizer and an additional sunscreen if applicable (Figure P14–4-25).

14 End the facial by washing your hands and quietly letting the client know you are finished. Give the client instructions for getting dressed. Have her come out to the reception area when ready to discuss the home-care products and regime (Figure P14-4-26).

Clean-Up and Sanitation

15 Discard all disposable supplies and materials.

16 Close product containers tightly, clean them, and put them away in their proper places. Return unused cosmetics and other clean items to the dispensary.

17 Place used towels, coverlets, head covers, and other linens in a closed, covered laundry hamper.

18 Disinfect your workstation, including the facial table.

19 Wash your hands with soap and warm water.

CAUTION!

For sanitary reasons, never remove products from containers with your fingers. Always use a spatula. Do not touch fingertips to lids or openings of containers.

FOCUS ON . . .

CLIENTS

The importance of following proper hygiene and sanitation guidelines when giving facials cannot be overemphasized. As much as possible, wash your hands in the presence of your clients. When they see you doing this, they will have more confidence in your sanitation procedures.

PROCEDURE 14–4: THE BASIC STEP-BY-STEP FACIAL

Rubrics are used in education for organizing and interpreting data gathered from observations of student performance. It is a clearly developed scoring document used to differentiate between levels of development in a specific skill performance or behavior. Rubrics are provided in this supplement for use as either a self-assessment tool to aid the student in behavior development or as an educator assessment tool to determine competence. Space is provided to record steps needed for further growth and improvement.

Rate performance according to the following scale:

1 **Development Opportunity:** There is little or no evidence of competency; Assistance is needed; Performance includes multiple errors.

2 **Fundamental:** There is beginning evidence of competency; Task is completed alone; Performance includes few errors.

3 **Competent:** There is detailed and consistent evidence of competency; Task is completed alone; Performance includes rare errors.

4 **Strength:** There is detailed evidence of highly creative, inventive, mature presence of competency.

Space is provided for comments to assist you in improving your performance and achieving a higher rating.

PERFORMANCE ASSESSED	1	2	3	4	IMPROVEMENT PLAN
Preparation					
1. Gathered equipment, supplies, disposables, and products.					
2. Set up room.					
3. Prepared the bed, equipment, and workstation.					
4. Helped client prepare for the service.					
5. Properly placed client's headband.					
Procedure					
1. Cleansed own hands.					
2. Applied warm towel to décolleté.					
3. Applied warm towel to face.					
Cleanse					
1. Removed eye makeup if applicable.					
2. Properly removed product with spatula (fingertips were never used).					
3. Applied cleanser to fingertips.					
4. Started at neck or décolleté and spread cleanser upward and outward on chin, jaws, cheeks, and temples.					
5. Spread cleanser down nose and along its sides and bridge.					
6. Made small, circular movements around nose.					
7. Cleansed brows, forehead, and temples.					
8. Cleansed neck and chest.					

PERFORMANCE ASSESSED	1	2	3	4	IMPROVEMENT PLAN
9. Cleansed both sides of face.					
10. Cleansed forehead, eye area, temples, and forehead.					
11. Removed cleanser starting at neck or forehead and followed facial contours.					
Skin Analysis					
1. Covered client's eyes with eye pads.					
2. Properly positioned magnifying light.					
3. Noted skin type, condition, and texture.					
Machine Steaming					
1. Preheated the steamer.					
2. Turned on ozone button if applicable.					
3. Positioned steamer 18" away from face.					
4. Steamed face for 5 to 10 minutes.					
5. Turned off steamer after use.					
Towel Steaming					
1. Checked and confirmed towel temperature.					
2. Applied steaming towels to face.					
3. Steamed with towels for 2 minutes.					
4. Performed extractions following steaming, if applicable.					
Massage					
1. Selected appropriate massage cream.					
2. Applied massage cream to face, neck, shoulders, and chest.					
3. Performed correct massage procedure.					
4. Removed massage cream using warm towels or cleansing pads.					
Mask					
1. Chose appropriate mask formula.					
2. Properly warmed and removed mask.					
3. Applied mask with fingers or brush starting at neck and using slow strokes from center of face, moving outward to sides.					
4. Continued applying mask on jawline and face from center outward.					
5. Avoided the eye area.					
6. Allowed mask to remain on face for 7 to 10 minutes.					
7. Removed mask with wet cotton pads, sponges, or towels.					
Tone and Moisturize					
1. Applied appropriate toner.					
2. Applied appropriate moisturizer.					

PERFORMANCE ASSESSED	1	2	3	4	IMPROVEMENT PLAN
Completion					
1. Washed own hands.					
2. Informed client service was complete and gave instructions for dressing.					
3. Discussed home-care products and regimen.					
Clean-Up and Sanitation					
1. Discarded all disposable supplies and materials.					
2. Closed product containers, cleaned, and stored properly.					
3. Placed used towels and other linens in covered hamper.					
4. Disinfected workstation and facial table.					
5. Washed own hands with soap and warm water.					

14-4

SUPPLIES
- cotton roll
- scissors
- basin of warm water
- product

Preparation

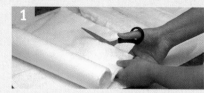

Prepare cotton. *(Figure P14–5-1)*

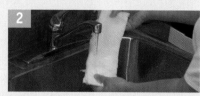

Wet and unfold the cotton strip. *(Figure P14–5-2)*

1 Prepare the cotton on an SMA (Figure P14–5-1).

2 Wet and unfold the cotton strip, and carefully divide it lengthwise into three separate strips (Figure P14–5-2). Try to keep the thickness of each strip as even as possible.

Procedure

The steps for applying a cotton compress alone or over a mask are as follows:

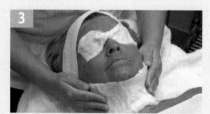

Take the strip that feels the thinnest and mold it to the client's neck. *(Figure P14–5-3)*

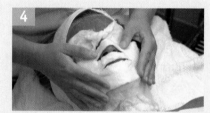

Apply the cotton under the jaw, chin, and lower part of the cheeks. *(Figure P14–5-4)*

3 Secure eye pads on the client's eyes. Take the strip that feels the thinnest and mold it to the client's neck. Be sure the strip does not overlap on the underside of the chin and jawline (Figure P14–5-3).

4 Place the center of the second strip of cotton (saving the thickest piece for last) on the chin, under the lower lip. Mold the cotton under the jaw, chin, and lower part of the cheeks. Leave breathing access by molding the strips around the tip of the nose (Figure P14–5-4).

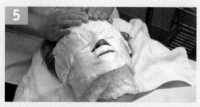

(Figure P14–5-5)

5 Place the third and thickest cotton strip over the upper portion of the face (eye pads remain in place). Carefully stretch the cotton (Figure P14–5-5).

PROCEDURE 14–5: APPLYING THE COTTON COMPRESS

Rubrics are used in education for organizing and interpreting data gathered from observations of student performance. It is a clearly developed scoring document used to differentiate between levels of development in a specific skill performance or behavior. Rubrics are provided in this supplement for use as either a self-assessment tool to aid the student in behavior development or as an educator assessment tool to determine competence. Space is provided to record steps needed for further growth and improvement.

Rate performance according to the following scale:

1 **Development Opportunity:** There is little or no evidence of competency; Assistance is needed; Performance includes multiple errors.

2 **Fundamental:** There is beginning evidence of competency; Task is completed alone; Performance includes few errors.

3 **Competent:** There is detailed and consistent evidence of competency; Task is completed alone; Performance includes rare errors.

4 **Strength:** There is detailed evidence of highly creative, inventive, mature presence of competency.

Space is provided for comments to assist you in improving your performance and achieving a higher rating.

14–5

PERFORMANCE ASSESSED	1	2	3	4	IMPROVEMENT PLAN
Preparation					
1. Gathered equipment, supplies, disposables, and products.					
2. Prepared the cotton.					
3. Wet cotton strip.					
4. Unfolded cotton strip.					
5. Divided cotton strip lengthwise into three separate strips.					
6. Maintained uniform thickness of strips.					
Procedure					
1. Secured eye pads on client's eyes.					
2. Molded cotton strip to client's neck.					
3. Did not overlap neck strip on the underside of chin and jawline.					
4. Placed center of second cotton strip on chin under lower lip.					
5. Molded cotton under jaw, chin, and lower part of cheeks.					
6. Molded strips around tip of nose to leave breathing access.					
7. Placed a cotton strip over the upper portion of the face.					
8. Used care in stretching cotton.					
9. Proceeded with service before removing the compress.					

1 *Optional step:* Massage over the surface of the compress mask with an ice cube or cool face globes if available, using circular movements. The ice will feel refreshing and will firm the skin. As the ice melts, the water seeps into the compress, helping to soften the mask underneath.

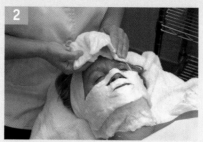

Slide the compress slowly toward the side of the face, picking up as much of the treatment mask as possible. *(Figure P14–6-1)*

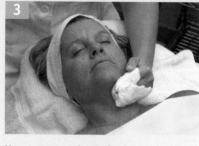

Use a cotton mitt to further remove remaining traces of the mask. *(Figure P14–6-2)*

2 Starting on the upper part of the face, place the hands, palms down, on each side of the face. With one hand, slide the compress slowly toward the side of the face, picking up as much of the treatment mask as possible (Figure P14–6-1). The eye pads will come off at the same time and should be discarded. Fold the strip in half, so that the side of the compress that has the treatment mask on it is inside and the compress strip has two clean surfaces. Squeeze the cotton over a waste container to remove any excess water.

3 Tear a separate strip of wet cotton in half, wrapping around the first three fingers of the hand to form a cotton mitt. Use a cotton mitt to further remove remaining traces of the mask (Figure P14–6-2). If necessary, cotton pads, rather than finger mitts, can be used to cleanse the face.

When all traces of the treatment mask have been removed, move down to the next cotton compress strip and repeat the same steps. Repeat again on the neck strip.

PROCEDURE 14–6: REMOVING THE COTTON COMPRESS

Rubrics are used in education for organizing and interpreting data gathered from observations of student performance. It is a clearly developed scoring document used to differentiate between levels of development in a specific skill performance or behavior. Rubrics are provided in this supplement for use as either a self-assessment tool to aid the student in behavior development or as an educator assessment tool to determine competence. Space is provided to record steps needed for further growth and improvement.

Rate performance according to the following scale:

1 **Development Opportunity:** There is little or no evidence of competency; Assistance is needed; Performance includes multiple errors.

2 **Fundamental:** There is beginning evidence of competency; Task is completed alone; Performance includes few errors.

3 **Competent:** There is detailed and consistent evidence of competency; Task is completed alone; Performance includes rare errors.

4 **Strength:** There is detailed evidence of highly creative, inventive, mature presence of competency.

Space is provided for comments to assist you in improving your performance and achieving a higher rating.

PERFORMANCE ASSESSED	1	2	3	4	IMPROVEMENT PLAN
Optional Step					
1. Massaged over surface of compress mask with ice cubes or cool face globes.					
Procedure					
1. At upper part of face, placed hands, palms down, on each side of face.					
2. Using one hand, slid the compress slowly toward side of face.					
3. Picked up as much of treatment mask as possible.					
4. Removed eye pads simultaneously.					
5. Discarded eye pads.					
6. Folded compress in half with treatment mask on the inside.					
7. Discarded compress.					
8. Tore a separate strip of wet cotton in half.					
9. Wrapped wet strip around first three fingers to form cotton mitt.					
10. Removed remaining traces of mask.					
11. Moved to next compress strip and repeated removal process.					
12. Moved to neck strip and repeated removal process.					
Completion					
1. Performed completion and clean-up steps according to Procedure 14-4.					

14–6

SUPPLIES

- basin of water
- cotton pads
- gloves
- astringent
- zip-lock plastic bag
- other appropriate facial supplies, products, and equipment

Preparation

Preparing the Fingers for Comedone Extractions

If you are using 4" × 4" or 2" × 2" premade pads, apply astringent to pads (without oversaturating them) and wrap around fingers. If you are not using 4 premade pads, prepare cotton as follows.

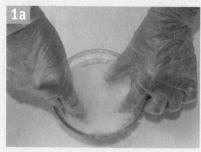 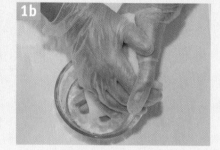

Wet cotton. *(Figure P14–7-1)*

1 Dip strips of clean cotton in water and squeeze out the excess (Figure P14–7-1a, b).

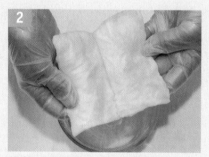 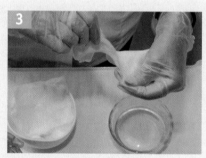

Divide pad in half. *(Figure P14–7-2)*　　Tear strips. *(Figure P14–7-3)*

2 Unfold the pad and divide it in half (Figure P14–7-2). Place one-half of the pad back in the bowl that holds the cleansing pads. With astringent, lightly saturate the half of the pad you are holding. Squeeze out the excess astringent.

3 Tear small strips from the astringent-saturated cotton (Figure P14–7-3).

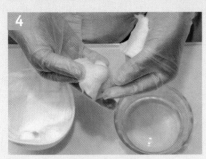

4 Put on gloves, and wrap fingers with dampened pads. Wrap the strips smoothly around the end of each index finger. Repeat this step until the fingertips are well padded (Figure P14–7-4).

Wrap strips around index fingers. *(Figure P14–7-4)*

Performing Extractions

Prepare the client's skin. Extractions are performed during a treatment after the skin is warmed and prepared/softened with product. Never extract on unprepared dry, cold skin. Extraction procedures for different facial areas follow:

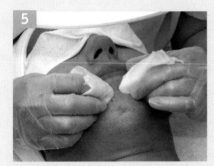

Extractions on the chin. *(Figure P14–7-5)*

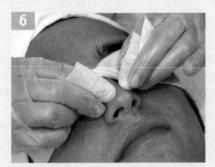

Extractions on the nose. *(Figure P14–7-6)*

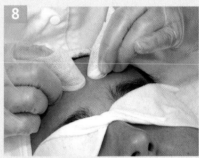

Extractions on the forehead. *(Figure P14–7-7)*

5 **Chin.** On a flat area, press down, under, and up. Work around the plug, pressing down, in, and up (Figure P14–7-5). Bring fingers in toward each other around the follicle without pinching.

6 **Nose.** Slide fingers down each side of the nose, holding the nostril tissue firmly, but do not press down too firmly on the nose. The fingers on top do the sliding, while the other one holds close to the bottom of the follicle. Do not cut off the air flow to the nostrils (Figure P14–7-6).

7 **Cheeks.** Slide fingers down the cheek, holding the skin as you go. The lower hand holds and the other hand slides toward the lower hand.

8 **Forehead; upper cheekbones.** Extract as on the chin: press down, in, and up (Figure P14-7-7).

14-7

Clean-Up and Sanitation

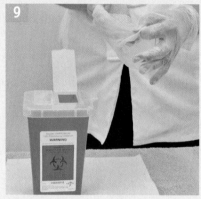

Change gloves. *(Figure P14-7-8)*

9 Dispose of gloves and supplies properly. Change gloves to continue the treatment (Figure P14-7-8).

10 After completing the treatment, perform the clean-up steps following a service. It is important to follow thorough sanitation procedures after doing extractions or an acne facial.

FYI

LANCETS

When a lesion is sealed over, as in old blackheads and closed comedones, a small-gauge needle or lancet is used for extraction. The lancet should be inserted at a 35-degree angle or parallel to the surface of the skin. Slowly insert the needle just under the top of the plug, lift the top off, and open it gently. Never put the needle down into the follicle because it is painful and could damage it. Extract in the appropriate direction to release sebum (Figure 14-20). Lancets are disposed of in biohazard containers.

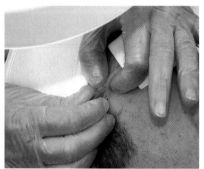

Using a lancet.

Rubrics are used in education for organizing and interpreting data gathered from observations of student performance. It is a clearly developed scoring document used to differentiate between levels of development in a specific skill performance or behavior. Rubrics are provided in this supplement for use as either a self-assessment tool to aid the student in behavior development or as an educator assessment tool to determine competence. Space is provided to record steps needed for further growth and improvement.

Rate performance according to the following scale:

1 **Development Opportunity:** There is little or no evidence of competency; Assistance is needed; Performance includes multiple errors.

2 **Fundamental:** There is beginning evidence of competency; Task is completed alone; Performance includes few errors.

3 **Competent:** There is detailed and consistent evidence of competency; Task is completed alone; Performance includes rare errors.

4 **Strength:** There is detailed evidence of highly creative, inventive, mature presence of competency.

Space is provided for comments to assist you in improving your performance and achieving a higher rating.

PERFORMANCE ASSESSED	1	2	3	4	IMPROVEMENT PLAN
Preparation					
1. Gathered equipment, supplies, disposables, and products.					
2. Set up room.					
3. Prepared the bed, equipment, and workstation.					
4. Helped client prepare for the service.					
5. Properly placed client's headband.					
6. Cleansed own hands.					
7. Applied gloves.					
8. If using premade pads, applied astringent to pads and wrapped around fingers.					
9. In the absence of premade pads, dipped strips of clean cotton in water and removed excess.					
10. Unfolded pad and divided in half.					
11. Placed one-half of pad in bowl that holds cleansing pads.					
12. Lightly saturated other half of pad with astringent.					
13. Squeezed out excess astringent.					
14. Tore small strips from the astringent-saturated cotton.					
15. Wrapped gloved index fingers with dampened pads.					

PERFORMANCE ASSESSED	1	2	3	4	IMPROVEMENT PLAN
Procedure					
1. Prepared client's skin.					
2. On flat chin area, pressed down, under, and up.					
3. Worked around plug, pressing down, in, and up.					
4. Brought fingers in toward each other around the follicle without pinching.					
5. Slid fingers down each side of nose, firmly holding nostril tissue.					
6. Did not press down too firmly on nose.					
7. Slid fingers down the cheek area, holding skin taut.					
8. Used same technique as on chin area for forehead and upper cheekbones.					
Clean-Up and Sanitation					
1. Disposed of gloves and supplies properly.					
2. Changed gloves to continue treatment.					
3. Performed clean-up steps found in Procedure 14–4.					

14–7

EQUIPMENT
- paraffin wax and heater

SUPPLIES
- paraffin wax brush
- covered trash container with plastic bag
- bowl
- spatula
- bolster
- disinfectant/sanitizer
- hand sanitizer/antibacterial soap

LINENS
- hand towels
- client gown or wrap
- clean linens
- blanket
- headband

DISPOSABLES
- gauze
- paper towels
- gloves
- cotton pads
- cotton rounds
- tissues

PRODUCTS
- cleanser
- serum
- mask
- toner
- eye cream
- moisturizer
- sunscreen
- lip balm

Preparation

1 Prepare the room and workstation for a facial.

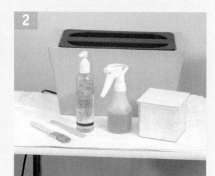

(Figure P14–8-1)

2 Melt the paraffin in a warming unit to a little more than body temperature (Figure P14–8-1). This may take an hour to heat up.

Procedure

3 Place eye pads on client.

4 Apply an appropriate product, such as a serum or hydrating mask, under the paraffin mask.

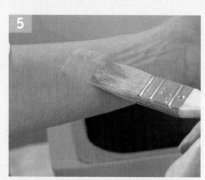

Test the temperature on the wrist.
(Figure P14–8-2)

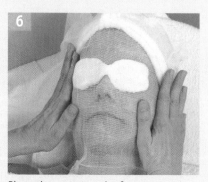

Place the gauze on the face.
(Figure P14–8-3)

5 Test the temperature of the paraffin on the wrist (Figure P14–8-2).

6 Cut the gauze to the desired size, and place it over the face and neck (Figure P14–8-3). It is not usually necessary to cut holes for the eyes and nose, because the gauze is woven very loosely. Occasionally, however, a client may feel claustrophobic. In that case, make slits in the gauze for the eyes, nose, and mouth. Precut gauze pads are available and are more efficient for this use.

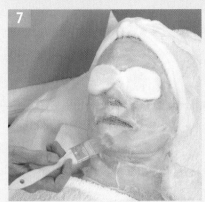

Apply the first coat of paraffin with a brush. *(Figure P14–8-4)*

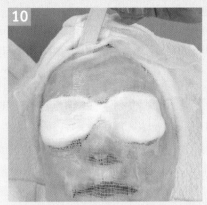

Use a wooden spatula to work the mask loose. *(Figure P14–8-5)*

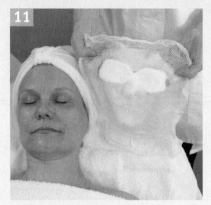

Carefully remove the mask. *(Figure P14–8-6)*

7 Apply the first coat of paraffin over the gauze with a brush, beginning at the base of the neck and working up to the forehead (Figure P14–8-4).

8 Continue adding layers of paraffin to the top of the gauze until the application is approximately ¼" thick. The application of wax will take several minutes.

9 After the wax application is completed, have the client relax until the wax is hardened and ready to remove (approximately 15 minutes).

10 When ready to remove the mask, use a wooden spatula to work the edges of the mask loose from the face and neck (Figure P14–8-5).

11 Carefully lift the mask from the neck in one piece (Figure P14–8-6).

12 Finish the service with the appropriate products (toner, moisturizer).

Clean-Up and Sanitation

13 Remove the head covering and show the client to the dressing room, offering assistance if needed.

14 Discard all disposable supplies and materials.

15 Close product containers tightly, clean them, and put them away in their proper places. Return unused cosmetics and other clean items to the dispensary.

16 Place used towels, head covers, and other linens in a closed, covered laundry hamper.

17 Disinfect supplies, equipment, and the workstation, including the facial table. Turn off the equipment.

18 Wash your hands with soap and warm water.

14–8

PROCEDURE 14–8: APPLYING THE PARAFFIN MASK

Rubrics are used in education for organizing and interpreting data gathered from observations of student performance. It is a clearly developed scoring document used to differentiate between levels of development in a specific skill performance or behavior. Rubrics are provided in this supplement for use as either a self-assessment tool to aid the student in behavior development or as an educator assessment tool to determine competence. Space is provided to record steps needed for further growth and improvement.

Rate performance according to the following scale:

1 **Development Opportunity:** There is little or no evidence of competency; Assistance is needed; Performance includes multiple errors.

2 **Fundamental:** There is beginning evidence of competency; Task is completed alone; Performance includes few errors.

3 **Competent:** There is detailed and consistent evidence of competency; Task is completed alone; Performance includes rare errors.

4 **Strength:** There is detailed evidence of highly creative, inventive, mature presence of competency.

Space is provided for comments to assist you in improving your performance and achieving a higher rating.

PERFORMANCE ASSESSED	1	2	3	4	IMPROVEMENT PLAN
Preparation					
1. Gathered equipment, supplies, disposables, and products.					
2. Set up room.					
3. Prepared the bed, equipment, and workstation.					
4. Helped client prepare for the service.					
5. Properly placed client's head covering.					
6. Melted paraffin in warming unit to little more than body temperature.					
Procedure					
1. Placed eye pads on client.					
2. Applied appropriate product (serum or hydrating mask).					
3. Tested temperature of paraffin on wrist.					
4. Cut gauze to desired size.					
5. Placed gauze over face and neck.					
6. Applied first coat of paraffin over gauze with brush.					
7. Began at neck and worked toward forehead.					
8. Continued adding paraffin until approximately ¼" thick.					
9. Allowed wax to harden for approximately 15 minutes.					
10. Used wooden spatula to work edges of mask loose from face and neck.					

PERFORMANCE ASSESSED	1	2	3	4	IMPROVEMENT PLAN
11. Carefully lifted mask from neck in one piece.					
12. Completed the service with the appropriate products (toner, moisturizer).					
Clean-Up and Sanitation					
1. Removed client's head covering.					
2. Escorted client to dressing room and offered assistance.					
3. Discarded disposable supplies and materials.					
4. Closed product containers, cleaned, and stored properly.					
5. Returned unused cosmetics and other clean items to dispensary.					
6. Placed used towels and other linens in covered hamper.					
7. Disinfected supplies, equipment, workstation, and facial table.					
8. Turned off equipment.					
9. Washed own hands with soap and warm water.					

14–8

SUPPLIES

- disinfectant/sanitizer
- hand towels
- hand sanitizer/antibacterial soap
- covered trash container
- bowls
- spatulas
- fan brush
- bolster
- blanket
- headband
- clean linens
- client gown or wrap

DISPOSABLES

- paper towels
- gloves/finger cots
- cotton pads/4" × 4" pads
- tissues
- cotton rounds
- plastic bag

PRODUCTS

- cleanser
- massage lotion
- toner
- moisturizer
- sunscreen

EQUIPMENT

- facial bed/table
- towel warmer (as needed)

The following procedure is a standard relaxing massage.

- Use a product that will easily glide across the skin. Warm the product before applying.
- A good rule of thumb is to repeat all movements consecutively three to six times.
- The number of movements to perform for each step may vary—these are only suggestions.
- Each instructor may have developed her or his own routine. Follow your instructors' lead.

Preparation

1 Set up the room.

2 Prepare the table, equipment, and workstation.

3 Help the client prepare for the service.

Procedure

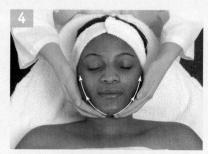

Apply the massage product with relaxing strokes. *(Figure P15–1–1)*

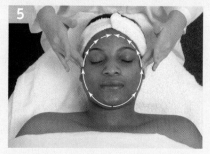

Move up to the forehead. *(Figure P15–1–2)*

4 With clean, warm hands, evenly apply the warmed massage product to the décolleté and face by using the hands or a soft brush (Figure P15–1–1). One teaspoon should be enough product for the facial area.

5 Start with hands on the décolleté (Figure P15–1–2). Move slowly up the sides of the neck and face to the forehead.

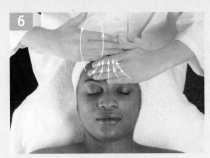

Begin upward strokes in the middle of the forehead and at the brow line. *(Figure P15–1-3)*

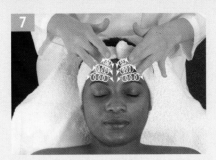

Begin a circular movement in the middle of the forehead along the brow line. *(Figure P15–1-4)*

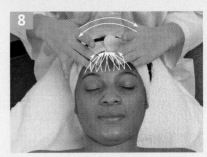

Start a crisscross stroking movement at the middle of the forehead, starting at the brow line. *(Figure P15–1-5)*

6 With the middle and ring fingers of each hand, start upward strokes in the middle of the forehead and at the brow line. Working upward toward the hairline, one hand follows the other as the hands move toward the right temple, move back across the forehead to the left temple, and then move back to the center of the forehead (Figure P15–1-3). Repeat the movements three to six times.

7 With the middle finger of each hand, start a circular movement in the middle of the forehead along the brow line. Continue this circular movement while working toward the temples. Bring the fingers back quickly to the center of the forehead at a point between the brow line and the hairline. Each time the fingers reach the temple, pause for a moment and apply slight pressure to the temple (Figure P15–1-4). Repeat three to six times.

8 With the middle and ring fingers of each hand, start a crisscross stroking movement at the middle of the forehead, starting at the brow line and moving upward toward the hairline. Move toward the right temple and back to the center of the forehead. Now move toward the left temple and back to the center of the forehead (Figure P15–1-5). Repeat three to six times.

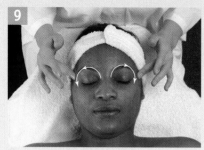

Slide the fingers to the outer corner of the eye, lifting the brow at the same time. *(Figure P15–1-6)*

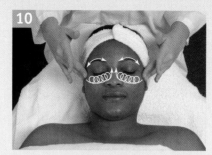

Start a circular movement at the outside corner of the eye, on the cheekbone to under the center of the eye. *(Figure P15–1-7)*

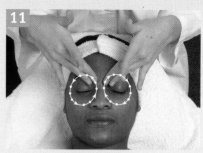

Tap lightly around the eyes. *(Figure P15–1-8)*

9 Place the ring fingers under the inside corners of the eyebrows and the middle fingers over the brows. Slide the fingers to the outer corner of the eye, lifting the brow at the same time (Figure P15–1-6). This movement continues with step 7.

10 Start a circular movement with the middle finger at the outside corner of the eye. Continue the circular movement on the cheekbone to the point under the center of the eye, and then slide the fingers back to the starting point (Figure P15–1-7). Repeat six to eight times. The left hand moves clockwise, and the right hand moves counterclockwise.

11 Start a light tapping movement with the pads of the fingers. Tap lightly around the eyes as if playing a piano. Continue tapping, moving from the temple, under the eye, toward the nose, up and over the brow, and outward to the temple. Do not tap the eyelids directly over the eyeball (Figure P15–1-8). Repeat six times.

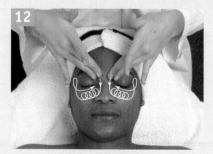

Begin a circular movement down the nose and continuing across the cheeks to the temples. *(Figure P15–1-9)*

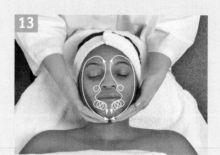

Begin a firm circular movement on the chin. *(Figure P15–1-10)*

12 With the middle finger of each hand, start a circular movement down the nose and continuing across the cheeks to the temples. Slide the fingers under the eyes and back to the bridge of the nose (Figure P15–1-9). Repeat the movements six times.

13 With the middle and ring fingers of each hand, slide the fingers from the bridge of the nose, over the brow (lifting the brow), and down to the chin. Start a firm circular movement on the chin with the thumbs. Change to the middle fingers at the corner of the mouth. Rotate the fingers five times, and slide the fingers up the

sides of the nose, over the brow, and then stop for a moment at the temple. Apply slight pressure on the temple. Slide the fingers down to the chin, and repeat the movements six times. The downward movement on the side of the face should have a very light touch to avoid dragging the skin downward (Figure P15–1-10).

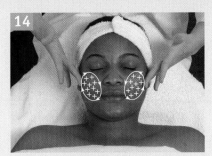

Begin a light tapping movement on the cheeks. *(Figure P15–1-11)*

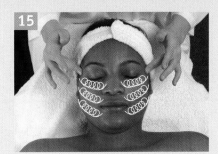

Begin a circular movement at the center of the chin and move up to the earlobes. *(Figure P15–1-12)*

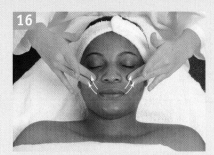

Begin the "scissor" movement. *(Figure P15–1-13)*

14 With the pads of the fingertips, start a light tapping movement (piano playing) on the cheeks, working in a circle around the cheeks (Figure P15–1-11). Repeat the movements six to eight times.

15 With the middle finger of each hand, start a circular movement at the center of the chin and move up to the earlobes. Slide the middle fingers to the corner of the mouth and then continue the circular movements to the middle of the ears. Return the middle fingers to the nose and continue the circular movements outward across the cheeks to the top of the ear (Figure P15–1-12). Repeat three to five times.

16 With the index and middle fingers of each hand, start the "scissor" movement, gliding from the center of the mouth, upward over the cheekbone, and stopping at the top of the cheekbone. Alternate the movement from one side of the face to the other, using the right hand on the right side of the face and then the left hand on the left side (Figure 15-1-13). Repeat eight to ten times.

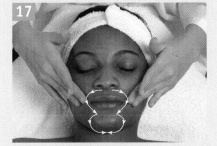

Draw the fingers from the center of the upper lip, around the mouth, under the lower lip, and under the chin. *(Figure P15–1-14)*

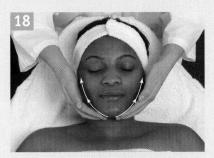

Begin a scissor movement from the center of the chin and then slide the fingers along the jawline to the earlobe. *(Figure P15–1-15)*

17 With the middle finger of both hands, draw the fingers from the center of the upper lip, around the mouth, under the lower lip, and then continue a circle under the chin (Figure 15-1-14). Repeat six to eight times.

18 With the index finger above the chin and jawline (the middle, ring, and little fingers should be under the chin and jaw), start a scissor movement from the center of the chin and then slide the fingers along the jawline to the earlobe. Alternate one hand after the other, using the right hand on the right side of the face and the left hand on the left side of the face (Figure P15–1-15). Repeat eight to ten times on each side of the face.

15–1

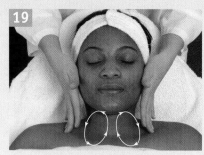

Apply light upward strokes over the front of the neck. *(Figure P15–1-16)*

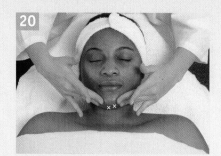

Tapping. *(Figure P15–1-17)*

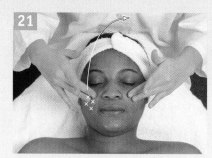

Tap and lift the cheek area. *(Figure P15–1-18)*

19 Apply light upward strokes over the front of the neck with both hands (Figure P15–1-16). Circle down and then back up, using firmer downward pressure on the outer sides of the neck. Repeat 10 times. Do not press down on the center of the neck.

20 With the middle and ring fingers of the right hand, give two quick taps under the chin, followed with one quick tap with the middle and ring fingers of the left hand. The taps should be done in a continuous movement, keeping a steady rhythm. The taps should be done with a light touch, but with enough pressure so that a soft tapping sound can be heard. Continue the tapping movement while moving the hands slightly to the right and then left, so as to cover the complete underside of the chin. Without stopping or breaking the rhythm of the tapping, move to the right cheek (Figure P15–1-17).

21 Continue the tapping on the right cheek in the same manner as under the chin, except the tapping with the left hand will have a lifting movement. The rhythm will be tap, tap, lift, tap, tap, lift, tap, tap, lift. Repeat this rhythmic movement 25 times. Without stopping the tapping movement, move the fingers back under the chin and over the left cheek, repeating the tapping and lifting movements. Move up and out on the area in a consistent pattern. Avoid tapping directly on the jawbone because this will feel unpleasant to the client (Figure P15–1-18).

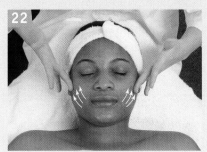

Begin a stroking movement at the mouth. *(Figure P15–1-19)*

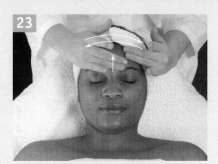

Move up to the outside corner of the left eye and across the forehead to the outside corner of the right eye. *(Figure P15–1-20)*

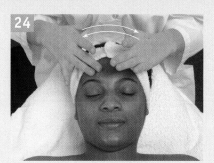

Let the movements grow slower, and feather off to end the massage. *(Figure P15–1-21)*

22 Without stopping the tapping movement, move back under the chin and over to the right corner of the mouth. Break into an upward, stroking movement with the first three fingers of each hand. One finger follows the other as each finger lifts the corner of the mouth. Repeat the movement 20 times. Continue the stroking movement as you quickly move under the chin to the left corner of the mouth (Figure P15–1-19). Repeat the stroking movement 20 times.

23 Without stopping the stroking movement, quickly move up to the outside corner of the left eye and continue the stroking, upward movement 20 times (Figure P15–1-20). Continue the stoking movement across the forehead to the outside corner of the right eye. Continue this stroking movement back and forth 20 times.

24 Continue the stroking movement back and forth across the fore-head, gradually slowing the move-ment. Let the movements grow slower and slower as the touch becomes lighter and lighter. Taper the movement off until the fin-gers are gradually lifted from the forehead (Figure P15–1-21). This slowing down of movement is often called "feathering."

25 Finish the service, and complete your client consultation.

Clean-Up and Sanitation

Follow appropriate facial clean-up and sanitation steps.

FYI

Blood returning to the heart from the head, face, and neck flows down the jugular veins on each side of the neck. All massage movements on the side of the neck are done with a downward (never upward) motion. Always slide gently upward in the center of the neck and circle out and then down on the sides.

15–1

Rubrics are used in education for organizing and interpreting data gathered from observations of student performance. It is a clearly developed scoring document used to differentiate between levels of development in a specific skill performance or behavior. Rubrics are provided in this supplement for use as either a self-assessment tool to aid the student in behavior development or as an educator assessment tool to determine competence. Space is provided to record steps needed for further growth and improvement.

Rate performance according to the following scale:

1 **Development Opportunity:** There is little or no evidence of competency; Assistance is needed; Performance includes multiple errors.

2 **Fundamental:** There is beginning evidence of competency; Task is completed alone; Performance includes few errors.

3 **Competent:** There is detailed and consistent evidence of competency; Task is completed alone; Performance includes rare errors.

4 **Strength:** There is detailed evidence of highly creative, inventive, mature presence of competency.

Space is provided for comments to assist you in improving your performance and achieving a higher rating.

PERFORMANCE ASSESSED	1	2	3	4	IMPROVEMENT PLAN
Preparation					
1. Gathered equipment, supplies, disposables, and products.					
2. Set up room.					
3. Prepared the bed, equipment, and workstation.					
4. Helped client prepare for the service.					
5. Properly placed client's headband.					
Procedure					
1. Cleansed own hands.					
2. Applied warm massage product to décolleté and face.					
3. Started at décolleté and moved slowly up sides of neck and face to the forehead.					
4. With middle and forefingers of both hands, applied upward strokes at the center of the forehead, moving to the outside temples and back to center.					
5. Repeated forehead movement three to six times.					
6. Applied circular movement with middle finger along the brow line and worked toward temples.					
7. Paused at the temples.					
8. Repeated three to six times.					
9. With middle and ring fingers, performed the crisscross stroking movement on forehead.					

PERFORMANCE ASSESSED	1	2	3	4	IMPROVEMENT PLAN
10. Repeated crisscross movement three to six times.					
11. Slid ring and middle fingers to the outer corner of the eye, lifting brow at the same time.					
12. Performed circular movement, using middle fingers, from the outside corner of the eye to under the center of the eye.					
13. Repeated six to eight times.					
14. Performed a light tapping movement around the eyes, moving from temples to under the eyes, toward the nose, up and over the brow, and outward to the temple.					
15. Began a circular movement down the nose and continued across the cheeks to the temples.					
16. Repeated movements six times.					
17. Began a circular movement down the nose and continuing across the cheeks to the temples.					
18. Repeated movement six times.					
19. Began a firm circular movement on the chin.					
20. Rotated fingers five times.					
21. Slid fingers up sides of nose, over brow, paused at temple, and applied pressure.					
22. Slid fingers down to chin.					
23. Repeated movement six times.					
24. Performed a light tapping movement on the cheeks, working in a circle around the cheeks.					
25. Repeated movement six to eight times.					
26. Began circular movement at center of chin and moved up to earlobes.					
27. Slid middle fingers to corner of mouth and continued circular movements to middle of ears.					
28. Returned middle fingers to nose and continued circular movements outward across cheeks to the top of ear.					
29. Repeated three to five times.					
30. Performed the "scissor" movement from center of mouth to top of cheekbones.					
31. Alternated scissor movement from one side of face to the other.					
32. Repeated movement eight to ten times.					
33. Drew fingers from center of upper lip, around mouth, under lower lip, and under chin.					
34. Repeated movement six to eight times.					

15–1

PERFORMANCE ASSESSED	1	2	3	4	IMPROVEMENT PLAN
35. Began a scissor movement at center of chin.					
36. Slid fingers along jawline to the earlobe.					
37. Repeated eight to ten times on each side of face.					
38. With both hands, applied light upward strokes over front of neck.					
39. Repeated movement ten times.					
40. Performed the tapping movement, keeping a steady rhythm.					
41. Continued tapping to lift the cheek area.					
42. Repeated rhythmic movement 25 times.					
43. Avoided tapping directly on the jawbone.					
44. Performed a stroking movement at the mouth.					
45. Repeated movement 20 times.					
46. Continued stroking movement under chin to corner of mouth.					
47. Repeated movement 20 times.					
48. Moved up to the outside corner of left eye and across forehead to outside corner of eyes.					
49. Repeated stroking movement 20 times.					
50. Continued stroking movement across forehead.					
51. Gradually slowed movements.					
52. Feathered off at end of massage.					
53. Completed service and client consultation.					
Clean-Up and Sanitation					
1. Washed own hands with soap and warm water.					
2. Informed client service was complete and gave instructions for dressing.					
3. Discussed home-care products and regimen.					
4. Discarded all disposable supplies and materials.					
5. Closed product containers, cleaned, and stored properly.					
6. Placed used towels and other linens in covered hamper.					
7. Disinfected workstation and facial table.					

PROCEDURE 17–1: EYEBROW TWEEZING

SUPPLIES

- towels
- tweezers
- cotton pads
- eyebrow brush
- emollient cream
- antiseptic lotion
- gentle eye makeup remover
- astringent
- disposable gloves
- station and sanitation supplies
- client release form and chart

Preparation

Set up the station and have the client sign the release form.

In preparing for the tweezing procedure, perform the following steps:

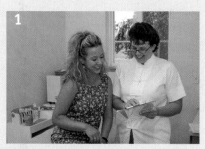

Discuss ideal eyebrow shape with client. *(Figure P17–1-1)*

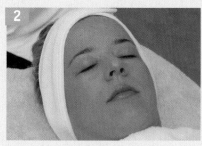

Seat and drape client. *(Figure P17–1-2)*

1 Discuss with the client the type of eyebrow arch suitable for his or her facial characteristics (Figure P17-1-1).

2 Seat the client in a facial chair in a reclining position, as for a facial massage. Or, if you prefer, seat the client in a half-upright position and work from the side (Figure P17-1-2).

3 Drape a towel over the client's clothing.

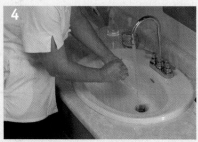

Wash hands. *(Figure P17–1-3)*

4 Wash and dry your hands, and put on disposable gloves. Washing your hands thoroughly with soap and warm water is critical before and after every client procedure you perform (Figure P17-1-3). The importance of proper sanitation in these procedures cannot be overemphasized.

Procedure

The eyebrow tweezing procedure involves the following steps:

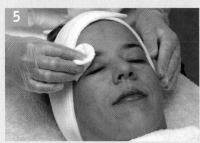

Apply a mild antiseptic before tweezing. *(Figure P17–1-4)*

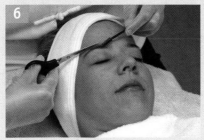

Trim long hairs outside the brow line. *(Figure P17–1-5)*

5 Use a mild antiseptic on a cotton pad before tweezing to clean and prepare the area (Figure P17-1-4).

6 Brush the eyebrows with a small brush. Carefully trim long hairs outside the brow line now or after tweezing (Figure P17–1-5). Brush the hair upward and into place to see the natural line of the brow.

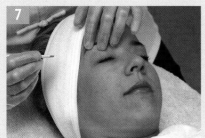

Stretch the skin taut with the index finger and thumb. *(Figure P17–1-6)*

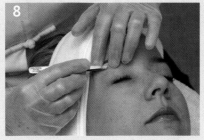

Remove hairs from below the brow line. Grasp each hair and pull with a quick, smooth motion. *(Figure P17–1-7)*

7 Stretch the skin taut with the index finger and thumb (or index and middle fingers) of your other hand (Figure P17–1-6).

8 Remove hairs from under the eyebrow line. Shape the lower section of one eyebrow; then shape the other. Grasp each hair individually with tweezers and pull with a quick, smooth motion in the direction of the hair growth (Figure P17–1-7). Grasp the hair at the base as close to the skin as possible without pinching the skin.

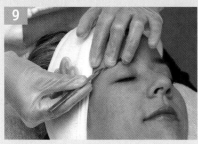

Remove stray hairs from above the brow line. *(Figure P17–1-8)*

9 Brush the hair downward. Remove hairs from above the eyebrow line (Figure P17–1-8). Shape the upper section of one eyebrow; then shape the other.

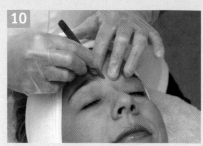

Remove hairs from between the eyebrows. *(Figure P17–1-9)*

10 Remove hair from between the brows (Figure P17–1-9).

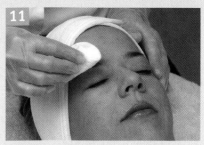

Apply an antiseptic lotion. *(Figure P17–1-10)*

11 Sponge the tweezed areas with a cotton pad, moistened with a nonirritating antiseptic lotion, to contract the skin and avoid infection (Figure P17–1-10).

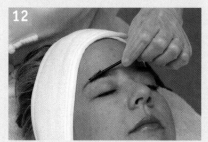

Brush eyebrow hair. *(Figure P17–1-11)*

12 Brush the eyebrow hair in its normal position (Figure P17–1-11).

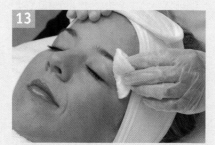

Apply soothing cream. *(Figure P17–1-12)*

13 *Optional:* Apply a soothing cream. Gently remove excess cream with a cotton pad (Figure P17–1-12).

14 Wash your hands with soap and warm water.

Clean-Up and Sanitation

15 Perform sanitation procedures. If eyebrow tweezing is part of a makeup or facial service, continue the procedure. If not, complete the next step.

16 Remove the towel from the client and place it in a closed hamper.

17 Accompany the client to the reception area and suggest rebooking. (The eyebrows should be tweezed about once a week.)

18 Discard disposable materials in a closed receptacle and disinfect the implements.

FYI

Always wash your hands before preparing and setting up for a service, after draping, and immediately after any service before walking the client out.

Rubrics are used in education for organizing and interpreting data gathered from observations of student performance. It is a clearly developed scoring document used to differentiate between levels of development in a specific skill performance or behavior. Rubrics are provided in this supplement for use as either a self-assessment tool to aid the student in behavior development or as an educator assessment tool to determine competence. Space is provided to record steps needed for further growth and improvement.

Rate performance according to the following scale:

1 **Development Opportunity:** There is little or no evidence of competency; Assistance is needed; Performance includes multiple errors.

2 **Fundamental:** There is beginning evidence of competency; Task is completed alone; Performance includes few errors.

3 **Competent:** There is detailed and consistent evidence of competency; Task is completed alone; Performance includes rare errors.

4 **Strength:** There is detailed evidence of highly creative, inventive, mature presence of competency.

Space is provided for comments to assist you in improving your performance and achieving a higher rating.

PERFORMANCE ASSESSED	1	2	3	4	IMPROVEMENT PLAN
Preparation					
1. Gathered equipment, supplies, disposables, and products.					
2. Set up room.					
3. Prepared the bed, equipment, and workstation.					
4. Discussed the suitable arch for the client's facial characteristics.					
5. Helped client prepare for the service.					
6. Properly placed client's headband.					
7. Draped towel over client's clothing.					
8. Washed and dried own hands.					
9. Put on disposable gloves.					
Procedure					
1. Prepared area by applying a mild antiseptic with a cotton pad.					
2. Brushed eyebrows with brow brush.					
3. Carefully trimmed long hairs outside brow line.					
4. Brushed hair upward and into place to see natural line of brow.					
5. Stretched the skin taut with index finger and thumb.					
6. Removed hairs from under the brow line.					
7. Shaped lower section of one eyebrow and then the other.					

17–1

PERFORMANCE ASSESSED	1	2	3	4	IMPROVEMENT PLAN
8. Grasped individual hair with tweezers and pulled with a quick, smooth motion in the direction of hair growth.					
9. Brushed brow hairs downward.					
10. Shaped upper section of one brow and then the other.					
11. Removed hair from between brows.					
12. Sponged tweezed areas with a cotton pad moistened with antiseptic lotion.					
13. Brushed eyebrow hair into normal placement.					
14. Optional: Applied a smoothing cream to area.					
15. Removed excess cream with a cotton pad.					
16. Proceeded with additional services as applicable.					
Clean-Up and Sanitation					
1. Discarded all disposable supplies and materials.					
2. Closed product containers, cleaned, and stored properly.					
3. Removed towel from client and placed used towels and other linens in covered hamper.					
4. Accompanied client to reception area.					
5. Suggested rebooking in one week.					
6. Disinfected workstation and facial table.					
7. Washed own hands with soap and warm water.					

SUPPLIES

- wax release form and chart
- facial chair
- high-level disinfectant
- roll of disposable paper or towels
- wax
- wax heater
- wax remover
- small disposable applicators or rollers
- fabric strips for hair removal and scissors
- hair cap or headband
- towels for draping
- disposable gloves
- plastic bag
- cotton pads and swabs
- powder
- surface cleaner (alcohol/oil)
- wax cleaning towel
- mild skin cleanser
- emollient or antiseptic lotion
- tweezers

This procedure for eyebrow waxing employs the use of a strip to remove soft wax. Adapt this procedure to all other body areas to be waxed.

Preparation

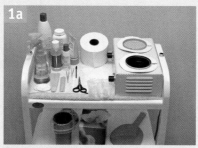 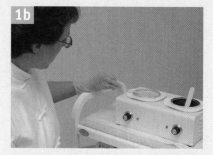

Prepare the wax. *(Figure P17–2-1a,b)*

1. Melt the wax in the heater. The length of time it takes to melt the wax depends on how full the wax holder is; approximately 20 minutes if it is full; 10 minutes if it is a quarter to half full. Be sure the wax is not too hot (Figure P17–2-1).

2. Complete the client consultation, release form, contraindications, and determine what hair you need to remove.

3. Lay a clean towel over the top of the facial chair and then a layer of disposable paper.

4. Place a hair cap or headband over the client's hair.

5. Drape a towel over the client's clothing as necessary.

6. Wash and dry your hands, and put on disposable gloves.

Procedure

The soft pot wax procedure with strips includes the following steps:

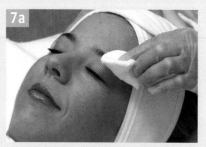 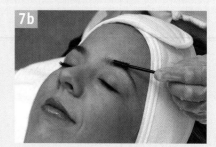

Cleanse the area thoroughly with a mild astringent cleanser, and dry. *(Figure P17-2-2)*

Brush the hair into place to see the brow line. *(Figure P17–2-3)*

7. Remove makeup. Cleanse the area thoroughly with a mild astringent cleanser, and dry (Figure P17-2-2). Apply a non-talc powder, if applicable. Brush the hair into place to see the brow line (Figure P17–2-3).

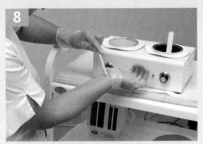

Test the temperature of the wax.
(Figure P17–2-4)

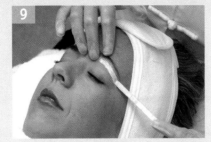

Spread a thin coat of wax evenly over the area. *(Figure P17–2-5)*

8 Test the temperature and consistency of the heated wax by applying a small drop on the inside of your wrist. It should be warm but not hot, and it should run smoothly off the spatula (Figure P17–2-4).

9 Wipe off one side of the spatula on the inside edge of the pot, so it does not drip. Carefully take it from the pot to the brow area. If it is dripping off the spatula, there is too much wax, or it is too hot. Correct the problem to avoid drips or hurting the client.

10 With the spatula or applicator, spread a thin coat of the warm wax evenly over the area to be treated, following the direction of the hair growth (Figure P17–2-5). Be sure not to put the spatula in the wax more than once (do not double-dip). Be sure not to use an excessive amount of wax, because it will spread when the fabric is pressed and may cover hair you do not wish to remove. Hold the skin taut near the edge where the wax is first applied.

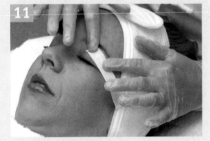

Apply a clean fabric strip over the area to be waxed. *(Figure P17–2-6)*

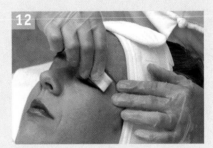

Hold the skin tight and remove the strip. *(Figure P17–2-7)*

11 Apply a clean fabric strip over the area to be waxed. Start the edge of the strip at the edge of the wax where you first applied it. Do not cover the rest of the brow with the strip. This way you can see the exposed area that you do not want to wax. Press gently in the direction of hair growth, running your finger over the surface of the fabric three to five times (Figure P17–2-6).

12 Gently but firmly hold the skin taut, placing the middle and ring fingers of one hand on either side of the strip as close as possible to where you will start to pull. Hold the loose edge of the strip at the end and quickly remove the fabric strip by pulling in the direction opposite to the hair growth. Do not lift or pull straight up on the strip; doing so could damage or remove the skin (Figure P17–2-7).

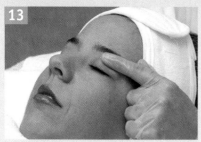

Apply pressure to the area after the wax strip is removed. *(Figure P17–2-8)*

13 Immediately apply pressure with your finger to the treated area. Hold it there for approximately five seconds to relieve the painful sensation (Figure P17–2-8).

14 Remove any excess wax residue from the skin with the cotton strip by gently lifting it sideways in the same direction as the hair growth. You can carefully remove excess wax without removing hairs this way.

15 Repeat the wax procedure on the area around the other eyebrow.

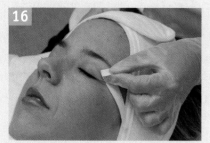

Remove excess wax residue. *(Figure P17–2-9)*

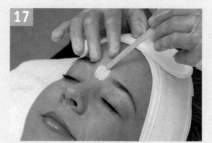

Wax between the brows. *(Figure P17–2-10)*

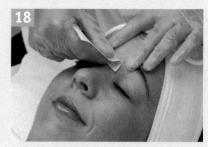

Pull the strip straight down. *(Figure P17–2-11)*

16 For the area between the brows, apply the wax (generally in an upward direction between the nose and the forehead). Line the bottom of the strip up to the bottom edge of the wax. Hold the skin tight on both sides of the strip above the brows with the middle and ring fingers. Hold the top of the strip and pull the strip straight down close to the nose without lifting. This can be done all in one section or in two halves—the right and the left (Figure P17–2-9).

17 Cleanse the skin with a mild wax remover, and apply a post-wax product or antiseptic lotion (Figure P17–2-10).

18 Tweeze the remaining stray hairs, and apply a cold compress if necessary. If it is too slippery or there is wax residue, apply the post-wax products after tweezing; or rinse the area with water and pat dry before tweezing.

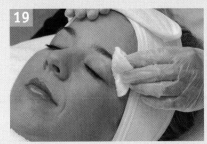

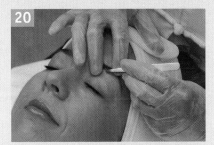

Cleanse the skin and apply an emollient or antiseptic lotion. *(Figure P17–2-12)*

Tweeze stray hairs. *(Figure P17–2-13)*

Finish all services with the client precautions and the post-consultation.

Follow all services with sanitation clean-up procedures.

Clean-Up and Sanitation for All Procedures

Remove the headband and towel drape from the client, and place them in a closed hamper.

Discard all used disposable materials in a closed waste container. Never reuse wax. Do not place the used spatula, muslin strips, wax, or any other materials used in waxing directly on the counter.

Wash your hands with soap and warm water.

Sanitize and disinfect the treatment area. This includes counter surfaces, the facial chair, the wax heater, the mag lamp, implements, containers, bottle caps/lids, and the floor.

CAUTION!

Never leave the wax heater on overnight because it is a fire hazard and can affect the quality of the wax.

17-2

Here's a Tip

Excess wax will get on the tweezers and interfere with tweezing. Remove all wax and post-products with a moist cotton pad before tweezing, and reapply soothing products after tweezing.

CAUTION!

If the wax strings and lands in an area you do not wish to treat, remove it with lotion designed to dissolve and remove wax. Do not apply the strip over any area that should not be waxed.

PROCEDURE 17–2: EYEBROW WAXING WITH SOFT WAX

Rubrics are used in education for organizing and interpreting data gathered from observations of student performance. It is a clearly developed scoring document used to differentiate between levels of development in a specific skill performance or behavior. Rubrics are provided in this supplement for use as either a self-assessment tool to aid the student in behavior development or as an educator assessment tool to determine competence. Space is provided to record steps needed for further growth and improvement.

Rate performance according to the following scale:

1 **Development Opportunity:** There is little or no evidence of competency; Assistance is needed; Performance includes multiple errors.

2 **Fundamental:** There is beginning evidence of competency; Task is completed alone; Performance includes few errors.

3 **Competent:** There is detailed and consistent evidence of competency; Task is completed alone; Performance includes rare errors.

4 **Strength:** There is detailed evidence of highly creative, inventive, mature presence of competency.

Space is provided for comments to assist you in improving your performance and achieving a higher rating.

PERFORMANCE ASSESSED	1	2	3	4	IMPROVEMENT PLAN
Preparation					
1. Gathered equipment, supplies, disposables, and products.					
2. Set up room.					
3. Prepared the bed, equipment, and workstation.					
4. Placed a clean towel over top of facial chair and covered it with a layer of disposable paper.					
5. Melted wax in heater for approximately 10 to 20 minutes.					
6. Completed client consultation, discussing contraindications and suitable arch for the client's facial characteristics.					
7. Properly placed client's headband.					
8. Draped towel over client's clothing.					
9. Washed and dried own hands.					
10. Put on disposable gloves.					
Procedure					
1. Prepared area by cleansing with a mild antiseptic with a cotton pad.					
2. Dried area thoroughly.					
3. Applied a non-talc powder.					
4. Brushed hair into place to see brow line.					
5. Tested temperature and consistency of wax.					
6. Dipped spatula in wax.					

PERFORMANCE ASSESSED	1	2	3	4	IMPROVEMENT PLAN
7. Took appropriate steps to prevent dripping.					
8. Spread a thin coat of warm wax over area to be treated, following direction of hair growth.					
9. Held skin taut near edge where wax was first applied.					
10. Applied fabric strip over area to be waxed.					
11. Did not cover rest of brow with strip.					
12. Pressed gently in direction of hair growth, running fingers over surface multiple times.					
13. Gently, but firmly, held the skin taut and quickly removed the fabric strip.					
14. Pulled the fabric strip in the direction opposite to hair growth.					
15. Applied pressure with fingers to treated area.					
16. Maintained pressure for 5 seconds.					
17. Removed excess wax residue from skin with cotton strip.					
18. Repeated procedure on other eyebrow.					
19. Applied wax between brows in an upward direction between nose and forehead.					
20. Lined up bottom edge of strip with bottom edge of wax application and applied.					
21. Held skin taut and pulled strip downward in one or two steps.					
22. Cleansed skin with a mild wax remover.					
23. Applied a post-wax product or antiseptic lotion.					
24. Tweezed remaining stray hairs.					
Clean-Up and Sanitation					
1. Discarded all disposable supplies and materials.					
2. Closed product containers, cleaned, and stored properly.					
3. Removed towel from client and placed used towels and other linens in covered hamper.					
4. Accompanied client to reception area.					
5. Suggested rebooking.					
6. Disinfected workstation and facial table.					
7. Washed own hands with soap and warm water.					

SUPPLIES

Use the same list of supplies as for the eyebrow waxing in Procedure 17–2.

Procedure

The lip waxing procedure with hard wax includes the following steps:

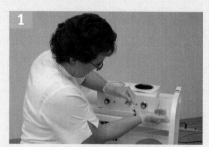

Test wax temperature. *(Figure P17–3-1)*

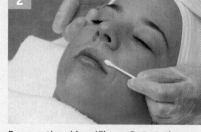

Prepare the skin. *(Figure P17–3-2)*

1 Prepare the client and test the temperature of the wax on your arm or wrist (Figure P17–3-1).

2 Prepare the skin (Figure P17–3-2). For lip waxing, have the client hold the lips tightly together to make waxing easier on the skin.

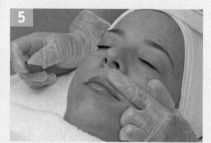

Apply wax to the upper lip, one side at a time, leaving a "tab or handle" to grasp. *(Figure P17–3-3)*

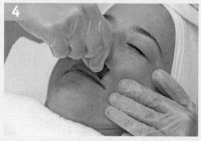

Pull off wax in the appropriate direction. *(Figure P17–3-4)*

3 Apply wax to one side of the upper lip outward from the center to the corner, leaving a "tab or handle" to grasp (Figure P17–3-3). (If using soft wax, apply the strip.)

4 Hold the skin tight, and quickly pull parallel to the skin without lifting up (Figure P17–3-4).

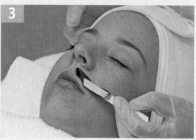

Apply pressure. *(Figure P17–3-5)*

5 Immediately apply pressure to the waxed area to ease any discomfort (Figure P17–3-5).

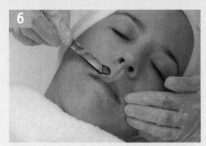

Repeat on other side. *(Figure P17–3-6)*

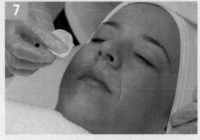

Apply soothing lotion. *(Figure P17–3-9)*

6 Repeat on the other side of the lip (Figure P17-3-6).

7 Apply after-wax soothing lotion (Figure P17-3-9).

8 Finish all services with the client precautions and the post-consultation.

9 Follow all services with sanitation clean-up procedures.

PROCEDURE 17–3: LIP WAXING PROCEDURE WITH HARD WAX

Rubrics are used in education for organizing and interpreting data gathered from observations of student performance. It is a clearly developed scoring document used to differentiate between levels of development in a specific skill performance or behavior. Rubrics are provided in this supplement for use as either a self-assessment tool to aid the student in behavior development or as an educator assessment tool to determine competence. Space is provided to record steps needed for further growth and improvement.

Rate performance according to the following scale:

1 **Development Opportunity:** There is little or no evidence of competency; Assistance is needed; Performance includes multiple errors.

2 **Fundamental:** There is beginning evidence of competency; Task is completed alone; Performance includes few errors.

3 **Competent:** There is detailed and consistent evidence of competency; Task is completed alone; Performance includes rare errors.

4 **Strength:** There is detailed evidence of highly creative, inventive, mature presence of competency.

Space is provided for comments to assist you in improving your performance and achieving a higher rating.

PERFORMANCE ASSESSED	1	2	3	4	IMPROVEMENT PLAN
Preparation					
1. Gathered equipment, supplies, disposables, and products.					
2. Set up room.					
3. Prepared the bed, equipment, and workstation.					
4. Placed a clean towel over top of facial chair and covered it with a layer of disposable paper.					
5. Melted wax in heater for approximately 10 to 20 minutes.					
6. Completed client consultation, discussing contraindications and suitable arch for the client's facial characteristics.					
7. Properly placed client's headband.					
8. Draped towel over client's clothing.					
9. Washed and dried own hands.					
10. Put on disposable gloves.					
Procedure					
1. Tested wax temperature.					
2. Prepared area and had client hold lips tightly together.					
3. Applied wax to one side of upper lip outward from center to corner.					
4. Held skin tight and quickly pulled wax parallel to skin.					
5. Immediately applied pressure to waxed area to ease discomfort.					

PERFORMANCE ASSESSED	1	2	3	4	IMPROVEMENT PLAN
6. Repeated procedure on other side of lip.					
7. Applied after-wax soothing lotion.					
8. Completed all other services as applicable.					
9. Completed post-consultation.					
Clean-Up and Sanitation					
1. Discarded all disposable supplies and materials.					
2. Closed product containers, cleaned, and stored properly.					
3. Removed towel from client and placed used towels and other linens in covered hamper.					
4. Accompanied client to reception area.					
5. Suggested rebooking.					
6. Disinfected workstation and facial table.					
7. Washed own hands with soap and warm water.					

17–3

SUPPLIES

Use the same list of supplies as for the eyebrow waxing in Procedure 17–2.

REGULATORY AGENCY ALERT

Some states or provinces require estheticians to (1) sanitize the skin before tweezing or waxing and (2) apply an antiseptic at the end of the procedure. Always check with your regulatory agency to be sure you are complying with its requirements.

Procedure

1 Test the wax.

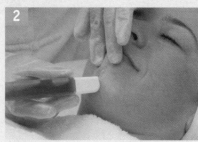

Apply the wax in small sections above the curve of the jawline. *(Figure P17–4-1)*

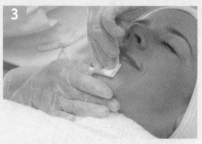

Hold the skin tight and pull opposite to the hair growth and parallel to the skin. *(Figure P17–4-2)*

2 Apply the wax in small sections above the curve of the jawline (Figure P17–4-1). Do not go over the curve. Wax above the jawline, then below it using separate pulls. Or you can wax below the jawline first, then above it.

3 Apply the strip, hold the skin tight, and pull opposite to the hair growth and parallel to the skin (Figure P17–4-2).

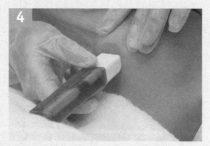

Apply the wax below the jawline. *(Figure P17-4-3)*

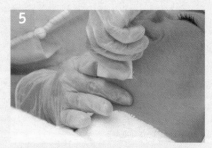

Hold the skin tight and pull opposite to the hair growth and parallel to the skin. *(Figure P17-4-4)*

4 Apply the wax in small sections below the curve of the jawline (Figure P17–4-3).

5 Apply the strip, hold the skin tight, and pull opposite to the hair growth and parallel to the skin (Figure P17–4-4).

6 Apply pressure if necessary without pressing hard on the throat or neck.

8 Finish all services with the client precautions and the post-consultation.

7 Finish the procedure.

9 Follow all services with sanitation clean-up procedures.

PROCEDURE 17-4: CHIN WAXING WITH SOFT WAX

Rubrics are used in education for organizing and interpreting data gathered from observations of student performance. It is a clearly developed scoring document used to differentiate between levels of development in a specific skill performance or behavior. Rubrics are provided in this supplement for use as either a self-assessment tool to aid the student in behavior development or as an educator assessment tool to determine competence. Space is provided to record steps needed for further growth and improvement.

Performance is evaluated according to the following scale:

1 **Development Opportunity:** There is little or no evidence of competency; Assistance is needed; Performance includes multiple errors.

2 **Fundamental:** There is beginning evidence of competency; Task is completed alone; Performance includes few errors.

3 **Competent:** There is detailed and consistent evidence of competency; Task is completed alone; Performance includes rare errors.

4 **Strength:** There is detailed evidence of highly creative, inventive, mature presence of competency.

Space is provided for comments to assist you in improving your performance and achieving a higher rating.

17-4

PERFORMANCE ASSESSED	1	2	3	4	IMPROVEMENT PLAN
Preparation					
1. Gathered equipment, supplies, disposables, and products.					
2. Set up room.					
3. Prepared the bed, equipment, and workstation.					
4. Placed a clean towel over top of facial chair covered by a layer of disposable paper.					
5. Melted wax in heater for approximately 10 to 20 minutes.					
6. Completed client consultation, discussing contraindications.					
7. Properly placed headband.					
8. Draped towel over client's clothing.					
9. Washed and dried own hands.					
10. Put on disposable gloves.					
Procedure					
1. Tested wax temperature					
2. Applied wax in small sections above the curve of the jawline.					
3. Applied strip.					
3. Held skin tight and pulled strip opposite to hair growth and parallel to skin.					
4. Applied pressure.					
5. Applied wax in small sections below curve of jawline.					

PERFORMANCE ASSESSED	1	2	3	4	IMPROVEMENT PLAN
6. Applied strip.					
7. Held skin tight and pulled strip opposite to hair growth and parallel to skin.					
8. Applied pressure.					
9. Completed the procedure.					
10. Completed all remaining services as applicable.					
Clean-Up and Sanitation					
1. Discarded all disposable supplies and materials.					
2. Closed product containers, cleaned, and stored properly.					
3. Removed towel from client and placed used towels and other linens in covered hamper.					
4. Accompanied client to reception area.					
5. Suggested rebooking.					
6. Disinfected workstation and facial table.					
7. Washed own hands with soap and warm water.					

17-4

SUPPLIES

Use the same list of supplies as for the eyebrow waxing in Procedure 17–2.

Procedure

Leg waxing can be started with either the front or the back of the legs. Visually divide the front of the legs in quarter sections (below the knees) and use a set pattern, starting removal at the bottom half of the lower legs. Make sure the skin is held tight, especially around the ankle, which is more sensitive.

1 Cleanse the area to be waxed with a mild astringent cleanser and dry. Apply a light dusting of powder if necessary.

2 Test the temperature and consistency of the heated wax.

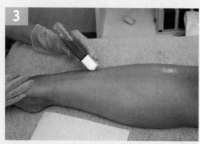

Apply the wax to the leg in a set pattern. *(Figure P17–5-1)*

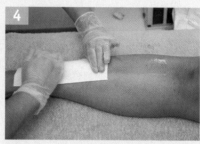

Apply the strip. *(Figure P17–5-2)*

3 Using a metal or disposable spatula or roller, spread a thin coat of warm wax evenly over the skin surface in the same direction as the hair growth (Figure P17–5-1).

4 Apply a fabric strip in the same direction as the hair growth. Press gently but firmly, running your hand over the surface of the fabric three to five times (Figure P17–5-2).

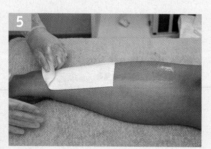

Hold the skin tight and remove the strip. *(Figure P17–5-3)*

5 Hold the skin taut with one hand close to where you will pull with the other hand, and quickly remove the wax in the opposite direction of the hair growth without lifting (Figure P17–5-3).

6 Quickly put your hand down to apply pressure to the treated area for approximately five seconds.

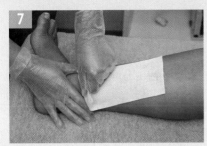

Repeat steps using fresh fabric strips.
(Figure P17–5-4)

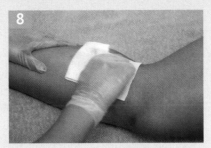

Repeat procedure on back of legs.
(Figure P17–5-5)

7 Repeat, taking a fresh fabric strip as each strip becomes too thick with wax (Figure P17–5-4).

8 Have the client turn over, and repeat the procedure on the backs of the legs (Figure P17–5-5).

9 Remove any remaining residue of wax from the skin, and apply an emollient or antiseptic lotion.

10 Finish all services with the client precautions and the post-consultation.

11 Follow all services with standard sanitation clean-up procedures.

Clean-Up and Sanitation

Follow these steps for leg waxing clean-up and sanitation:

12 Discard used disposable materials in a closed waste container.

13 Place linens and robe in a closed hamper.

14 Remove any wax from the metal spatula (if you used one) with wax removal solution. Disinfect the spatula and store it in a clean, covered container.

15 Disinfect the equipment, treatment bed, implements, waxer, and counters/surfaces.

16 Wash your hands.

Here's a Tip

If skin is too dry or cold, wax may stick and may not come off properly.

PROCEDURE 17–5: LEG WAXING PROCEDURE WITH SOFT WAX

Rubrics are used in education for organizing and interpreting data gathered from observations of student performance. It is a clearly developed scoring document used to differentiate between levels of development in a specific skill performance or behavior. Rubrics are provided in this supplement for use as either a self-assessment tool to aid the student in behavior development or as an educator assessment tool to determine competence. Space is provided to record steps needed for further growth and improvement.

Rate performance according to the following scale:

1 **Development Opportunity:** There is little or no evidence of competency; Assistance is needed; Performance includes multiple errors.

2 **Fundamental:** There is beginning evidence of competency; Task is completed alone; Performance includes few errors.

3 **Competent:** There is detailed and consistent evidence of competency; Task is completed alone; Performance includes rare errors.

4 **Strength:** There is detailed evidence of highly creative, inventive, mature presence of competency.

Space is provided for comments to assist you in improving your performance and achieving a higher rating.

PERFORMANCE ASSESSED	1	2	3	4	IMPROVEMENT PLAN
Preparation					
1. Gathered equipment, supplies, disposables, and products.					
2. Set up room.					
3. Prepared the bed, equipment, and workstation.					
4. Melted wax in heater for approximately 10 to 20 minutes.					
5. Completed client consultation; discussed contraindications.					
6. Washed and dried own hands.					
7. Put on disposable gloves.					
Procedure					
1. Cleansed area with mild astringent cleanser and dried.					
2. Applied light dusting of powder.					
3. Tested wax temperature and consistency.					
4. Used metal or disposable spatula or roller to spread a thin coat of warm wax evenly over skin surface in direction of hair growth.					
5. Applied fabric strip in same direction of hair growth.					
6. Pressed gently but firmly, running hand over surface of fabric three to five times.					
7. Held skin taut with one hand while removing wax in opposite direction of hair growth.					

PERFORMANCE ASSESSED	1	2	3	4	IMPROVEMENT PLAN
8. Applied pressure to treated area for about 5 seconds.					
9. Repeated waxing steps using fresh fabric as needed.					
10. Removed any remaining residue of wax.					
11. Applied an emollient or antiseptic lotion.					
12. Completed all services and post-consultation.					
Clean-Up and Sanitation					
1. Discarded all disposable supplies and materials.					
2. Closed product containers, cleaned, and stored properly.					
3. Removed wax from metal spatula with wax removal solution.					
4. Disinfected spatula and stored in clean, covered container.					
5. Accompanied client to reception area.					
6. Suggested rebooking.					
7. Disinfected workstation and facial table.					
8. Washed own hands with soap and warm water.					

17-5

PROCEDURE 17–6: UNDERARM WAXING PROCEDURE WITH HARD WAX

SUPPLIES

Use the same list of supplies as for the eyebrow waxing in Procedure 17–2.

Procedure

Because the hair under the arms grows in several different directions, it is important to first determine the number of different growth patterns and then to wax in sections following those patterns. Cut strips to the appropriate size if using soft wax. Divide the underarm area into approximately three sections or as hair growth patterns allow.

1 Wearing gloves, cleanse and sanitize the underarm area.

2 Apply a small amount of powder to the area to dry the area and facilitate the adherence of wax.

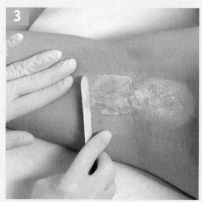

Apply wax to the first section of the underarm area. *(Figure P17–6-1)*

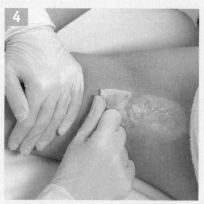

Grasp the wax edge or strip and pull against the hair growth. *(Figure P17–6-2)*

3 Apply wax to the first growth area, usually on the top or outer edge of the underarm. (Figure P17–6-1).

4 Grasp the wax "handle" or strip and quickly pull (Figure P17–6-2). Hold the skin tight when removing the wax.

5 Apply pressure immediately after wax removal to ease any pain.

6 Repeat the procedure on the next growth area—the bottom or inner edge of the underarm (Figure P17–6-3).

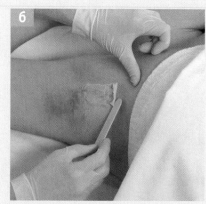

Repeat the procedure in the next area. *(Figure P17–6-3)*

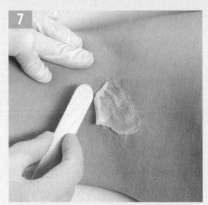

7

Repeat the procedure in the center of the underarm area. *(Figure P17–6-4)*

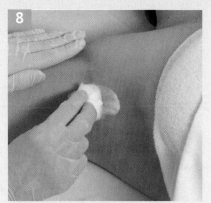

8

Apply a soothing after-wax lotion to calm any sensitivity. *(Figure P17–6-5)*

7 Repeat the procedure on the last growth area, or the center of the underarm (Figure P17-6-4). Remove any other stray hairs. Check in with the client to make sure she is comfortable and can handle any tweezing. It is a sensitive area, so the faster the procedure, the better.

8 Apply a soothing after-wax lotion; cold compresses are also nice to soothe the skin (Figure P17-6-5).

9 Finish with the client precautions and the post-consultation.

10 Perform sanitation clean-up procedures.

FOCUS ON . . .

THE CLIENT

Be mindful of your client's modesty. Try to make her as relaxed as possible, and do not expose the bikini area any more than she is comfortable with.

CAUTION!

When using hard wax, start with the lower sections of hair to apply the end section or "handle" of wax without hair underneath it. Each section then has a bare area at the bottom to form the next handle of the wax. Avoid pulling the hair underneath when first lifting the edge to grasp onto—it is very uncomfortable to lift the hair underneath with the wax stuck on it.

17-6

PROCEDURE 17–6: UNDERARM WAXING PROCEDURE WITH HARD WAX

Rubrics are used in education for organizing and interpreting data gathered from observations of student performance. It is a clearly developed scoring document used to differentiate between levels of development in a specific skill performance or behavior. Rubrics are provided in this supplement for use as either a self-assessment tool to aid the student in behavior development or as an educator assessment tool to determine competence. Space is provided to record steps needed for further growth and improvement.

Rate performance according to the following scale:

1 **Development Opportunity:** There is little or no evidence of competency; Assistance is needed; Performance includes multiple errors.

2 **Fundamental:** There is beginning evidence of competency; Task is completed alone; Performance includes few errors.

3 **Competent:** There is detailed and consistent evidence of competency; Task is completed alone; Performance includes rare errors.

4 **Strength:** There is detailed evidence of highly creative, inventive, mature presence of competency.

Space is provided for comments to assist you in improving your performance and achieving a higher rating.

PERFORMANCE ASSESSED	1	2	3	4	IMPROVEMENT PLAN
Preparation					
1. Gathered equipment, supplies, disposables, and products.					
2. Set up room.					
3. Prepared the bed, equipment, and workstation.					
4. Melted wax in heater for approximately 10 to 20 minutes.					
5. Completed client consultation; discussed contraindications.					
6. Washed and dried own hands.					
7. Put on disposable gloves.					
Procedure					
1. Cleansed and sanitized underarm area.					
2. Applied light dusting of powder.					
3. Tested wax temperature and consistency.					
4. Applied wax to first growth area.					
5. Held skin taut, grasped wax, and quickly pulled to remove.					
6. Applied pressure immediately to ease discomfort.					
7. Repeated procedure on remaining growth areas.					
8. Removed stray hairs.					
9. Applied a soothing after-wax lotion or cold compresses.					
10. Completed client post-consultation.					

PERFORMANCE ASSESSED	1	2	3	4	IMPROVEMENT PLAN
Clean-Up and Sanitation					
1. Discarded all disposable supplies and materials.					
2. Closed product containers, cleaned, and stored properly.					
3. Removed wax from metal spatula with wax removal solution.					
4. Disinfected spatula and stored in clean, covered container.					
5. Accompanied client to reception area.					
6. Suggested rebooking.					
7. Disinfected workstation and facial table.					
8. Washed own hands with soap and warm water.					

17-6

SUPPLIES

Use the same list of supplies as for the eyebrow waxing in Procedure 17–2.

Preparation

Prepare the station and the client. Always wear gloves.

Procedure

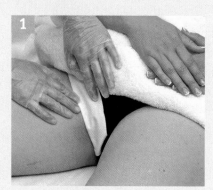

Drape the client. *(Figure P17–7-1)*

1 Tuck in a paper towel or wax strip along the edge of the client's bikini line. Cleanse and sanitize the area (Figure P17–7-1).

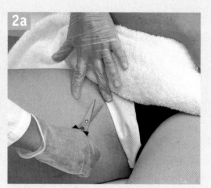

Trim the hair to ½ to ¾ of an inch. *(Figure P17–7-2)*

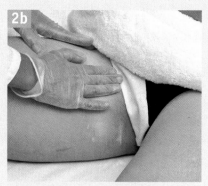

Apply powder. *(Figure P17–7-3)*

2 Trim the hair to ½" to ¾" in length if necessary (Figure P17–7-2). Apply a small amount of powder (Figure P17–7-3).

3 Bend the client's knee with the leg facing out. This position assists in reaching the inner bikini area and stretches the skin tighter. Be confident in moving the client's body position around to reach the right angle for waxing, but make sure the client is comfortable in the different positions.

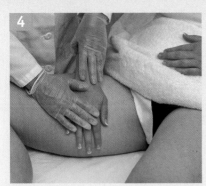

Show client where to place her hands.
(Figure P17–7-4)

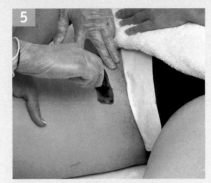

Apply wax above the curve. *(Figure P17–7-5)*

4 Have the client hold her skin tight next to the area being waxed. Show her where to place her hand and make sure that it is not in the way of the parallel pull (Figure P17–7-4).

5 Apply wax to the first growth area, usually on the upper, outer edge of the bikini line (Figure P17–7-5).

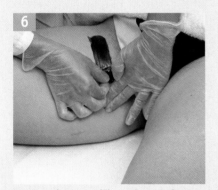

Remove the wax. *(Figure P17–7-6)*

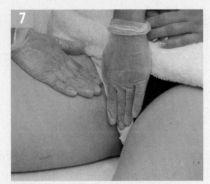

Apply pressure. *(Figure P17–7-7)*

6 Hold the skin tight, grasp the wax "handle," and quickly pull (Figure P17–7-6). Pull back parallel to the skin.

7 Apply pressure immediately to alleviate any discomfort (Figure P17–7-7).

17-7

Here's a Tip

When waxing sensitive areas such as underarms or bikini lines, trim the hair with scissors if it is more than ½" (1.25 cm) long.

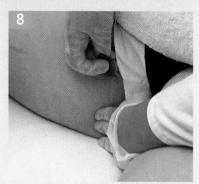

Work in sections. *(Figure P17–7-8)*

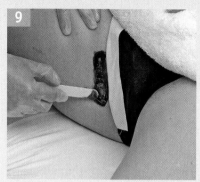

Apply wax below the curve. *(Figure P17–7-9)*

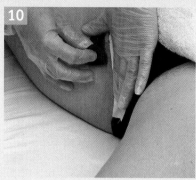

Remove the wax. *(Figure P17–7-10)*

8 Work in and down to the femoral ridge in sections. Do not wax over the curve of the femoral ridge (tendon). Wax the underside and the back side of the bikini area in separate sections (Figure P17–7-8).

9 To reach the back of the bikini area, have the client lift her leg toward her chest, grasping the ankle if possible. This also holds the skin tight (Figure P17–7-9).

10 Apply the wax and remove it without lifting (Figure P17–7-10).

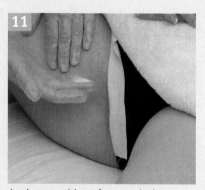

Apply a soothing after-wax lotion. *(Figure P17–7-11)*

11 Apply a soothing after-wax lotion (Figure P17–7-11). (Cold compresses are nice to soothe the skin.)

12 Finish all services with the client precautions and the post-consultation.

13 Perform sanitation clean-up procedures.

CAUTION!

Never go over the curve of the femoral ridge. Wax the top and bottom of the bikini area separately.

FYI

Brazilian waxing is an "extreme" bikini wax during which all of the hair is removed. Waxing procedures are the same; however, hard wax must be used, and the skin must be held tight because the area is so sensitive. Get advanced training in this technique before attempting it on clients.

PROCEDURE 17–7: BIKINI WAXING PROCEDURE WITH HARD WAX

Rubrics are used in education for organizing and interpreting data gathered from observations of student performance. It is a clearly developed scoring document used to differentiate between levels of development in a specific skill performance or behavior. Rubrics are provided in this supplement for use as either a self-assessment tool to aid the student in behavior development or as an educator assessment tool to determine competence. Space is provided to record steps needed for further growth and improvement.

Rate performance according to the following scale:

1 **Development Opportunity:** There is little or no evidence of competency; Assistance is needed; Performance includes multiple errors.

2 **Fundamental:** There is beginning evidence of competency; Task is completed alone; Performance includes few errors.

3 **Competent:** There is detailed and consistent evidence of competency; Task is completed alone; Performance includes rare errors.

4 **Strength:** There is detailed evidence of highly creative, inventive, mature presence of competency.

Space is provided for comments to assist you in improving your performance and achieving a higher rating.

PERFORMANCE ASSESSED	1	2	3	4	IMPROVEMENT PLAN
Preparation					
1. Gathered equipment, supplies, disposables, and products.					
2. Set up room.					
3. Prepared the bed, equipment, and workstation.					
4. Melted wax in heater for approximately 10 to 20 minutes.					
5. Completed client consultation, discussed contraindications.					
6. Washed and dried own hands.					
7. Put on disposable gloves.					
Procedure					
1. Tucked paper towel or wax strip along edge of client's bikini line.					
2. Cleansed area with mild astringent cleanser and dried.					
3. Trimmed hair to ½" to ¾" in length if necessary.					
4. Applied light dusting of powder.					
5. Bent client's knee with leg facing out.					
6. Made sure client was comfortable.					
7. Placed client's hands to hold skin taut.					
8. Applied wax to first growth area.					
9. Held skin taut.					
10. Grasped wax and quickly pulled back parallel to skin.					

17-7

PERFORMANCE ASSESSED	1	2	3	4	IMPROVEMENT PLAN
11. Applied pressure to minimize discomfort.					
12. Worked in and down to femoral ridge in sections.					
13. Waxed underside and back side of bikini area in separate sections.					
14. Had client lift leg toward chest.					
15. Applied wax and removed it without lifting.					
16. Applied a soothing after-wax lotion or cold compresses.					
17. Completed all services and post-consultation.					
Clean-Up and Sanitation					
1. Discarded all disposable supplies and materials.					
2. Closed product containers, cleaned, and stored properly.					
3. Removed wax from metal spatula with wax removal solution.					
4. Disinfected spatula and stored in clean, covered container.					
5. Accompanied client to reception area.					
6. Suggested rebooking.					
7. Disinfected workstation and facial table.					
8. Washed own hands with soap and warm water.					

17-7

SUPPLIES

Use the same list of supplies as for the eyebrow waxing in Procedure 17–2.

Waxing of the back and neck is a common procedure for many men. First determine the number of different growth patterns, and then wax in sections following those patterns. Do not wax large areas at one time. Leg strip sections are generally too large. Cut the leg strips to three-fourths of the length. Save the leftover part of the strip for other body parts. Have the client lie face down and start at the lower back area working up to the shoulders. Then have the client sit up for the top of the shoulder area if necessary. This procedure demonstrates a partial shoulder wax.

Procedure

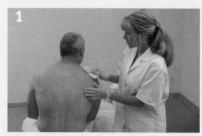

Sanitize the area. *(Figure P17–8-1)*

1. Cleanse and sanitize the area (Figure P17–8-1).

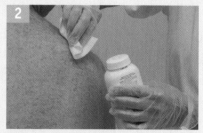

Apply powder. *(Figure P17–8-2)*

2. Apply a small amount of powder (Figure P17–8-2).

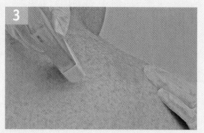

Apply the wax. *(Figure P17–8-3)*

3. Apply wax to the first growth area (Figure P17–8-3).

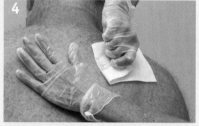

Remove the wax. *(Figure P17–8-4)*

4. Grasp the strip and quickly pull against the hair growth (Figure P17–8-4).

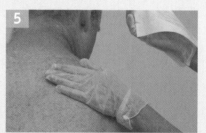

Apply pressure. *(Figure P17–8-5)*

5. Apply pressure immediately after wax removal to ease any pain (Figure P17–8-5).

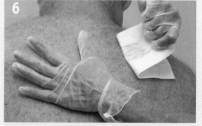

Repeat procedure. *(Figure P17–8-6)*

6. Repeat the procedure until all hair is removed (Figure P17–8-6).

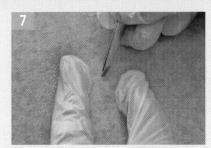

Remove stray hairs. *(Figure P17–8-7)*

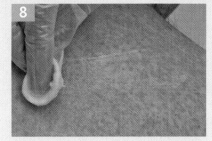

Apply soothing after-wax lotion. *(Figure P17–8-8)*

7 Remove any other stray hairs (Figure P17–8-7). Check in with the client to make sure he is comfortable. It is a sensitive area, so the faster the procedure, the better.

8 Apply a soothing after-wax lotion; cold compresses are also nice to soothe the skin (Figure P17–8-8).

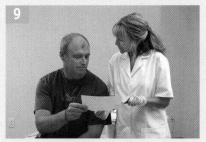

Client consultation. *(Figure P17–8-9)*

9 Clean-up and consultation: Remember to give your client post-wax precautions (Figure P17–8-9).

Here's a Tip

To wax a male client's shoulder and neck area, have him sit up and do the work from behind him.

17–8

PROCEDURE 17–8: MEN'S WAXING PROCEDURE WITH SOFT WAX

Rubrics are used in education for organizing and interpreting data gathered from observations of student performance. It is a clearly developed scoring document used to differentiate between levels of development in a specific skill performance or behavior. Rubrics are provided in this supplement for use as either a self-assessment tool to aid the student in behavior development or as an educator assessment tool to determine competence. Space is provided to record steps needed for further growth and improvement.

Rate performance according to the following scale:

1 Development Opportunity: There is little or no evidence of competency; Assistance is needed; Performance includes multiple errors.

2 Fundamental: There is beginning evidence of competency; Task is completed alone; Performance includes few errors.

3 Competent: There is detailed and consistent evidence of competency; Task is completed alone; Performance includes rare errors.

4 Strength: There is detailed evidence of highly creative, inventive, mature presence of competency.

Space is provided for comments to assist you in improving your performance and achieving a higher rating.

PERFORMANCE ASSESSED	1	2	3	4	IMPROVEMENT PLAN
Preparation					
1. Gathered equipment, supplies, disposables, and products.					
2. Set up room.					
3. Prepared the bed, equipment, and workstation.					
4. Melted wax in heater for approximately 10 to 20 minutes.					
5. Completed client consultation; discussed contraindications.					
6. Determined number of different growth patterns.					
7. Cut leg strips to three-fourths of the length.					
8. Had client lie face down.					
9. Washed and dried own hands.					
10. Put on disposable gloves.					
Procedure					
1. Cleansed area with mild astringent cleanser and dried.					
2. Applied light dusting of powder.					
3. Tested wax temperature and consistency.					
4. Used metal or disposable spatula or roller to spread a thin coat of warm wax evenly over skin surface in direction of hair growth.					
5. Applied fabric strip in same direction of hair growth.					

PERFORMANCE ASSESSED	1	2	3	4	IMPROVEMENT PLAN
6. Pressed gently but firmly, running hand over surface of fabric three to five times.					
7. Held skin taut with one hand while removing wax and strip in opposite direction of hair growth.					
8. Applied pressure to strips for about 5 seconds.					
9. Pulled strip opposite to hair growth and parallel to skin.					
10. Applied pressure.					
11. Removed any stray hairs.					
12. Repeated steps using fresh fabric strips.					
13. Removed any remaining waxy residue.					
14. Applied an emollient or antiseptic lotion.					
15. Completed all services and post-consultation.					
Clean-Up and Sanitation					
1. Discarded all disposable supplies and materials.					
2. Closed product containers, cleaned, and stored properly.					
3. Removed wax from metal spatula with wax removal solution.					
4. Disinfected spatula and stored in clean, covered container.					
5. Accompanied client to reception area.					
6. Suggested rebooking.					
7. Disinfected workstation and facial table.					
8. Washed own hands with soap and warm water.					

17-8

SKIN CARE PRODUCTS
- cleanser
- toner
- moisturizer

MAKEUP
- concealer
- highlighter
- contour color
- foundation
- powder
- eye shadow
- eyeliner
- mascara
- blush
- lip gloss
- lip liner
- lipstick

SUPPLIES
- cape
- disinfectant
- tweezers
- hair clip/headband
- brushes
- pencil sharpener
- mirror
- lash comb
- lash curler

DISPOSABLES
- spatulas
- cotton swabs
- mascara wands
- sponges
- tissues
- applicators

Your instructor may prefer a different method that may be equally correct. Completing a makeup application includes the consultation, setup, application, and clean-up procedures (Tables 19–10 and 19–11). Some artists like to apply the makeup working from the top to the bottom of the face—eyes, cheeks, and then lips. There are pros and cons to every method. You will likely come up with your own application procedure when working as a makeup artist.

Preparation

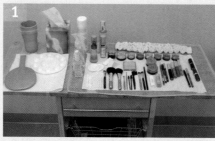

Set up products and colors. *(Figure P19–1-1)*

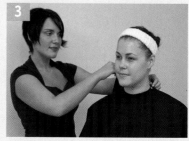

Drape the client. *(Figure P19–1-2)*

1 Determine the client's needs, and choose products and colors accordingly (Figure P19–1-1). Focus on your client's features and preferences. Discussing skin care or waxing is appropriate with a makeup client. Ask the following questions:
- Do you wear contacts or have allergies?
- What look do you want?
- What makeup products do you normally wear?
- What are your typical clothing colors?
- What is the special occasion or event?

2 Wash your hands.

3 Drape the client and use a headband or hair clip to keep her hair out of her face (Figure P19-1-2).

Procedure
Basic Makeup Applications

Preparing the face is like preparing a painting canvas for the palette of colors. The skin needs to be exfoliated and hydrated for the makeup to be applied successfully.

4   *Cleanser.* After washing your hands, cleanse the face if the client is wearing makeup or if the skin is oily.

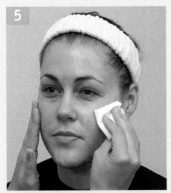

Apply toner or witch hazel. *(Figure P19–1-3)*

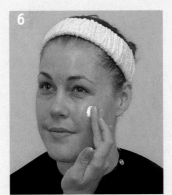

Apply moisturizer. *(Figure P19–1-4)*

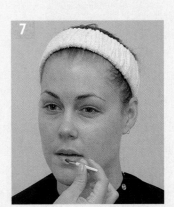

Lip conditioner. *(Figure P19–1-5)*

5   *Toner.* Use a cotton pad to apply the toner or witch hazel to cleanse the skin (Figure P19–1-3).

6   *Moisturizer.* Apply a moisturizer to prepare the skin for makeup (Figure P19–1-4).

7   *Lip conditioner.* Use a spatula to get the product out of the container. Apply with a brush (Figure P19–1-5). To give it more time to soak in and moisturize, put on the lip conditioner when starting the makeup application.

Note: Always use creams and liquids before applying powders, or they will not blend. If you are using a powder concealer or contour powder, apply these after the foundation.

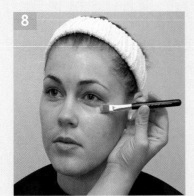

Apply the concealer. *(Figure P19–1-6)*

8   *Concealer.* Use a spatula to get the product out of the container. Choose a color one to two shades lighter than the foundation. You can apply this under or over the foundation beneath the eyes with a brush, sponge, or finger (Figure P19–1-6). It can also be used as the highlighter.

19–1

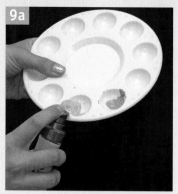

Choose the foundation. *(Figure P19–1–7)*

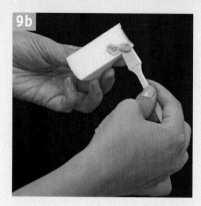

9 *Foundation.* Choose two colors to match the right shade. Use a spatula to get the product out of the container, or put some on a clean sponge or in a small container (Figure P19–1-7a,b). Apply to the jawline to match the skin color (Figure P19–1-8). Cover the skin to even out the skin tone and cover imperfections without over-rubbing the skin. Blend along the jaw and edges of the face (Figure P19–1-9). Blend downward to blend with facial hair and up around the hairline so the product does not stick in the hairline.

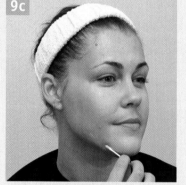

Apply to the jawline. *(Figure P19–1–8)*

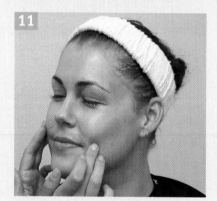

Blend the foundation. *(Figure P19–1-9)*

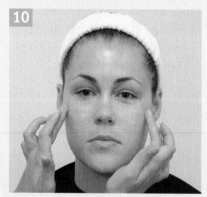

Apply highlighter to bring out features. *(Figure P19–1-10)*

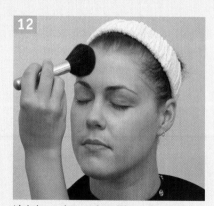

Apply contour for shading and minimizing features. *(Figure P19–1-11)*

Lightly apply powder. *(Figure P19–1-12)*

10 *Highlighter.* Use a spatula to get the product out of the container. Apply a white or light color to accentuate and bring out features along the brow bone, the temples, chin, or above the cheek bones. Blend with your brush, a sponge, or your finger (Figure P19–1-10).

11 *Contouring.* Use a spatula to get the product out of the container. Apply a darker shade under the cheekbones and to other features you want to appear smaller (Figure P19–1-11).

12 *Powder.* Pour a little powder on a tissue to avoid cross-contamination. Apply to the brush and tap off excess powder onto the tissue. Use a powder brush or puff, and sweep downward all over the face to set the foundation (Figure P19–1-12).

13

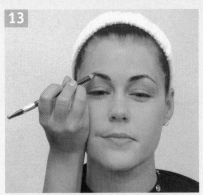

Color the brows using a pencil or brow powder. *(Figure P19–1-13)*

13 *Eyebrows.* Use a shade that is close to the hair color, or a shade the client likes. Apply color by using a pencil or cake eye shadow with a brush (Figure P19–1-13). Smudge with your finger, going in the opposite direction of the hair growth to blend. Then smooth back into place with a brow brush.

14a

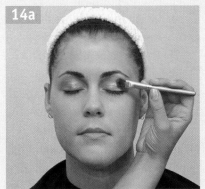

Apply the eye shadow base or light color all over the eye area. *(Figure P19–1-14)*

14b

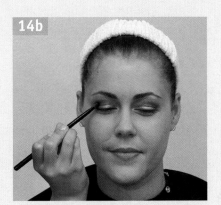

Apply a small amount of the darker eye shadow. *(Figure P19–1-15)*

14c

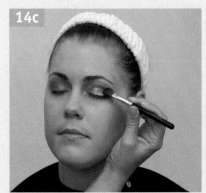

Blend the dark shadow. *(Figure P19–1-16)*

14 *Eye shadow.* Choose a light base color and apply all over the eyelid, from the lash line up to the brow. Stop color at the outside corner of the eye up to the outside corner of the brow (Figure P19–1-14).

Apply a darker shade to the crease: partially on top of the crease and partially underneath the crease. First tap the excess powder off the brush. Apply the color from the outside corner of

the eye to the area above the inside of the iris (Figure P19–1-15). Blend the color (Figure P19–1-16). *Optional:* Apply the eyeliner before applying the dark shadow color.

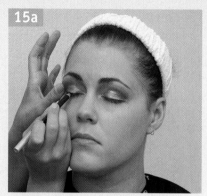

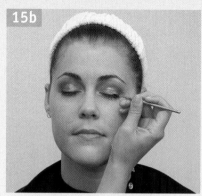

Line the eyes. *(Figure P19–1-17)*

Blend and set the liner. *(Figure P19-1-18)*

15 *Eyeliner.* Sharpen the liner before and after use. Wet liner can also be used with a disposable or sanitized brush. Eye shadow can be applied as liner with a thin brush dipped in water; dry shadow can also be applied with a thin, firm brush for a more natural look. Make sure the liner is not too rough or so dry that it drags on the eye.

Have the client shut her eyes when you apply the liner on top of the eyelids. Then have her look up and away as you apply the lower liner under the eyes (Figure P19–1-17).

Apply to the top and bottom edge of the eye on the outside of the lashes. Bring the liner three-fourths of the way to the center of the eye, ending softly at the inside of the iris. Blend so that the color tapers off. Bringing the liner closer to the nose can make the eyes appear closer together. Lining only the outside corner makes the eyes appear farther apart. Blend the liner with a firm, small liner brush (Figure P19–1-18).

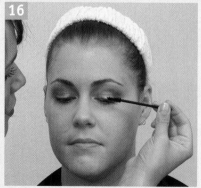

Carefully apply the mascara. *(Figure P19–1-19)*

16 *Mascara.* Dip a disposable brush into the mascara. Wipe off the excess. Have the client look down and focus on a fixed point to apply mascara to the top of the lashes (Figure P19-1-19). Comb with a lash comb before the product dries. Then have the client put her chin down while looking up at the ceiling to apply mascara to the bottom lashes. Comb before the client looks down to avoid smudging under the eye.

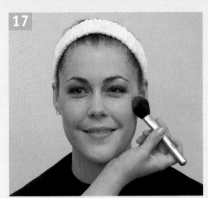

17

Apply the blush on the cheekbones. *(Figure P19–1-20)*

17 *Blush.* The blush color will depend on whether you choose a warm or cool color scheme. Tap off the excess powder on the brush. Apply blush just below the cheekbones, blending on top of the bones toward the top of the cheeks. The color should stop below the temple and not be closer than two fingers away from the nose. It should not go lower than the nose, because this can "drag down the face." Blush should blend to the hairline, but not into it. Do not apply too much blush on the apple of the cheek; this makes the face look fatter. A horizontal line makes the face appear wider, whereas a vertical line makes it look thinner. Following the cheekbones usually works best (Figure P19–1-20).

18 *Optional: Lip conditioner/lip gloss.* This step applies if you did not already apply lip moisturizer in step 4. Use a spatula to get the product out of the container. Use a brush to apply. Put on a gloss or lip moisturizer when starting the makeup application,

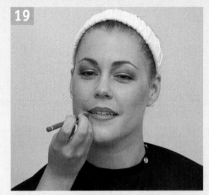

19

Line the lips. *(Figure P19–1-21)*

so it can soak in and moisturize before you start applying the liner. If the lips have too much gloss, the liner will not stick.

19 *Lip liner.* Sharpen the liner. Have the client smile and stretch her lips. With the lips pulled tight, the liner and lipstick brush glide on more smoothly. Line the outer edges of the lips first; then fill in and use the liner as a lipstick (Figure P19–1-21). This keeps the lipstick and color on longer.

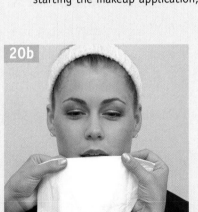

20a

Apply and blend lipstick. *(Figure P19–1-22)*

20b

Blot lipstick. *(Figure P19–1-23)*

20 *Lipstick.* Use a spatula to get the product out of the container. Have the client select a color from among two or three choices. Apply the lipstick evenly with a lip brush. Rest your ring finger on the client's chin to steady your hand. Ask the client to relax her lips and part them slightly. Brush on the lip color. Then ask the client to smile slightly so that you can smooth the lip color into any small crevices (Figure P19-1-22). Blot the lips with tissue to remove excess product and set the lip color (Figure P19-1-23).

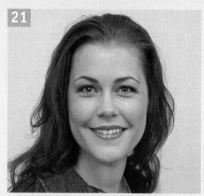

The finished look. *(Figure P19–1-24)*

21 Show the client the finished application (Figure P19-1-24).

Clean-Up and Sanitation

After the service is completed (and before the clean-up), fill out the client chart and make retail product suggestions and sales.

22 Wash your hands.

23 Discard all disposable items, such as sponges and applicators.

24 Disinfect implements such as eyelash curlers and tweezers.

25 Clean and disinfect brushes.

26 Place washable items in the laundry.

27 Disinfect product containers, used supplies, and the workstation.

FYI

Blending is the key to a professional makeup application.

Rubrics are used in education for organizing and interpreting data gathered from observations of student performance. It is a clearly developed scoring document used to differentiate between levels of development in a specific skill performance or behavior. Rubrics are provided in this supplement for use as either a self-assessment tool to aid the student in behavior development or as an educator assessment tool to determine competence. Space is provided to record steps needed for further growth and improvement.

Rate performance according to the following scale:

1 Development Opportunity: There is little or no evidence of competency; Assistance is needed; Performance includes multiple errors.

2 Fundamental: There is beginning evidence of competency; Task is completed alone; Performance includes few errors.

3 Competent: There is detailed and consistent evidence of competency; Task is completed alone; Performance includes rare errors.

4 Strength: There is detailed evidence of highly creative, inventive, mature presence of competency.

Space is provided for comments to assist you in improving your performance and achieving a higher rating.

PERFORMANCE ASSESSED	1	2	3	4	IMPROVEMENT PLAN
Preparation					
1. Gathered equipment, supplies, disposables, and products.					
2. Set up room.					
3. Prepared the bed, equipment, and workstation.					
4. Helped client prepare for the service.					
5. Performed consultation and determined client's needs.					
6. Chose colors.					
7. Cleansed own hands.					
8. Draped client and placed headband.					
Procedure					
1. Cleansed client's face.					
2. Applied toner using cotton pad.					
3. Applied moisturizer.					
4. Applied lip conditioner with a brush.					
5. Applied concealer with sponge, brush, or finger.					
6. Chose the correct foundation shade.					
7. Applied to jawline to match the skin tone.					
8. Covered the skin to even out skin tone and cover imperfections.					
9. Blended along jaw and edges of face.					
10. Blended downward and up and around hairline.					

19–1

115

PERFORMANCE ASSESSED	1	2	3	4	IMPROVEMENT PLAN
11. Applied a white or light color to accentuate and bring out features along brow bone, temples, chin, or above cheekbones.					
12. Blended with brush, sponge, or fingers.					
13. Applied contour for shading and minimizing features.					
14. Applied powder to brush and tapped off excess.					
15. Used powder brush or puff to sweep downward all over face to set the foundation.					
16. Enhanced brows by using pencil or cake eye shadow with a brush.					
17. Smudged shadow with finger.					
18. Chose light base eye shadow color and applied all over eyelid from lash line to brow.					
19. Applied a darker shade to the crease from the outside corner of the eye to the area above the inside of the iris.					
20. Sharpened liner before use.					
21. Applied liner on the upper lid from the outside of the eye toward the center of the eye as appropriate for how close set the eyes are.					
22. Applied liner on the lower lid in a similar manner.					
23. Blended liner with a firm, small liner brush.					
24. Dipped disposable brush into mascara and wiped off excess.					
25. Applied mascara to top of lashes.					
26. Combed with lash comb before product dried.					
27. Applied mascara to bottom of lashes.					
28. Combed with lash comb before product dried.					
29. Applied blush to cheekbones as appropriate for face shape.					
30. Sharpened lip liner.					
31. Applied lip liner to outer edges of the lips.					
32. Filled in and used liner as a lipstick.					
33. Applied lipstick evenly with a lip brush.					
34. Blotted lips with tissue to remove excess product and set lip color.					
35. Showed the client the finished application.					

PERFORMANCE ASSESSED	1	2	3	4	IMPROVEMENT PLAN
Clean-Up and Sanitation					
1. Washed own hands.					
2. Discarded all disposable supplies and materials.					
3. Disinfected implements.					
4. Cleaned and disinfected brushes.					
5. Placed washable items in the laundry.					
6. Disinfected product containers, used supplies, and workstation.					

SUPPLIES

- headband or hair clip
- tweezers
- eyelash comb/brush
- eyelash curler
- hand mirror
- small (manicure) scissors
- adjustable light
- adhesive tray or foil to put adhesive on
- makeup cape
- trays of artificial eyelashes

PRODUCTS

- eyelid and eyelash cleanser
- lash adhesive
- eyelash adhesive remover
- eye makeup remover
- hand sanitizer

DISPOSABLES

- cotton swabs
- cotton pads
- toothpick or hairpin
- mascara wand

Preparation

The following steps should be performed in preparation for applying artificial eyelashes.

1   Discuss with the client the desired length of the lashes and the effect she hopes to achieve.

2   Wash your hands.

3   Place the client in the makeup chair with her head at a comfortable working height. The client's face should be well and evenly lit; avoid shining the light directly into the eyes. Work from behind or to the side of the client. Avoid working directly in front of the client whenever possible.

4   Prepare for the makeup procedure, if applicable.

5   If the client wears contact lenses, she must remove them before starting the procedure.

6   If the client is only having artificial lashes applied and you have not already done so, remove mascara so that the lash adhesive will adhere properly. Work carefully and gently. Follow the manufacturer's instructions carefully.

Note: If the artificial lash application is in conjunction with a makeup application, complete the makeup without applying mascara to the lashes, and then finish with the false lashes.

Procedure

7   Brush the client's eyelashes to make sure they are clean and free of foreign matter, such as mascara particles (unless this is part of a makeup application). If the client's lashes are straight, they can be curled with an eyelash curler before you apply the artificial lashes.

8   Carefully remove the eyelash band from the package.

9   Start with the upper lash. If it is too long to fit the curve of the upper eyelid, trim the outside edge. Use your fingers to bend the lash into a horseshoe shape to make it more flexible so it fits the contour of the eyelid.

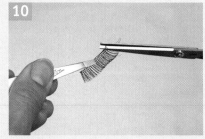

Feather the lashes with scissors. (*Figure P19–2–1*)

10   Feather band lashes to make uneven lengths on the end ("w" shapes) by nipping into it with the points of your scissors. This creates a more natural look (Figure P19–2–1).

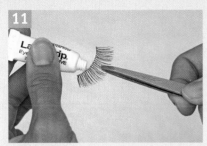
Apply adhesive to false lashes. *(Figure P19–2-2)*

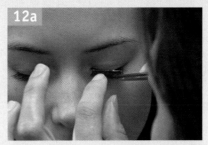
Apply lashes to the base of the natural lash line. *(Figure P19–2-3)*

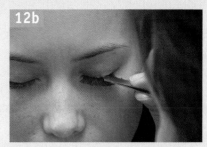
Press the lash on with an implement. *(Figure P19–2-4)*

11 Apply a thin strip of lash adhesive to the base of the false lashes with a toothpick or hairpin and allow a few seconds for it to set (Figure P19–2-2).

12 Apply the lashes by holding the ends with the fingers or tweezers.

For band lashes: Start with the shorter part of the lash and place it on the inner corner of the eye, toward the nose (Figure P19–2-3). Position the rest of the artificial lash as close to the client's own lash as possible.

For individual lashes: Apply five or six lashes, evenly spacing each one across the lash line. Use longer lashes on the outer edges of the eye, medium in the middle, and small on the inside by the nose.

Use the rounded end of a lash liner brush, a hairpin, or tweezers to press the lash on (Figure P19–2-4). Be very careful and gentle when applying the lashes. If eyeliner is to be used, the line is usually drawn on the eyelid before the lash is applied and retouched when the artificial lash is in place.

13 Apply the lower lash, if desired. Lower lash application is optional; it tends to look more unnatural. Trim the lash as necessary, and apply adhesive in the same way you did for the upper lash. Place the lash on top or beneath the client's lower lash. Place the shorter lash toward the center of the eye and the longer lash toward the outer part.

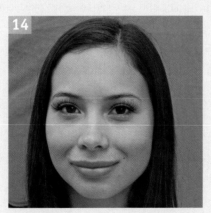
The finished look. *(Figure P19–2-5)*

14 Check the finished application and make sure the client is comfortable with the lashes (Figure P19–2-5). Remind the client to take special care with artificial lashes when swimming, bathing, or cleansing the face. Water, oil, or cleansing products will loosen artificial lashes. Band lash application lasts one day and are meant to be removed nightly. Individual lashes may last longer.

Clean-Up and Sanitation

15 Discard all disposable items.

16 Disinfect implements, such as the eyelash curler.

17 Clean and sanitize brushes using a commercial brush sanitizer.

18 Place all towels, linens, and the makeup cape in a laundry hamper.

19 Disinfect product containers, supplies, and the workstation.

20 Wash your hands with soap and warm water.

ACTIVITY

Examine industry journals or women's magazines:

- Find five pictures of makeup looks that you like and five that you dislike.
- Find one of each: natural, business, evening, and dramatic looks.
- Find a brow look you like and one you dislike.
- What is in style right now for makeup? Present an example in class.
- Find two professional articles about applying makeup.
- Make index cards with the list of supplies and the makeup application outline to refer to while practicing.

Rubrics are used in education for organizing and interpreting data gathered from observations of student performance. It is a clearly developed scoring document used to differentiate between levels of development in a specific skill performance or behavior. Rubrics are provided in this supplement for use as either a self-assessment tool to aid the student in behavior development or as an educator assessment tool to determine competence. Space is provided to record steps needed for further growth and improvement.

Rate performance according to the following scale:

1 **Development Opportunity:** There is little or no evidence of competency; Assistance is needed; Performance includes multiple errors.

2 **Fundamental:** There is beginning evidence of competency; Task is completed alone; Performance includes few errors.

3 **Competent:** There is detailed and consistent evidence of competency; Task is completed alone; Performance includes rare errors.

4 **Strength:** There is detailed evidence of highly creative, inventive, mature presence of competency.

Space is provided for comments to assist you in improving your performance and achieving a higher rating.

PERFORMANCE ASSESSED	1	2	3	4	IMPROVEMENT PLAN
Preparation					
1. Gathered equipment, supplies, disposables, and products.					
2. Set up room.					
3. Prepared the chair, equipment, and workstation.					
4. Helped client prepare for the service.					
5. Performed consultation and determined client's needs and desired lash length.					
6. Cleansed own hands.					
7. Seated client in makeup chair.					
8. Had client remove contact lenses, if applicable.					
9. Removed mascara.					
Procedure					
1. Brushed client's eyelashes to remove foreign matter.					
2. Carefully removed eyelash band from package.					
3. Trimmed band from outside edge to fit the eyelid.					
4. Shaped lash band to the contour of the eyelid.					
5. Point-cut the lash ends to create a more natural look.					
6. Applied a thin strip of lash adhesive to the band with a toothpick or hairpin and allowed a few seconds to set.					

PERFORMANCE ASSESSED	1	2	3	4	IMPROVEMENT PLAN
7. Applied band lashes by holding ends with fingers or tweezers, beginning with inner corner and working outward.					
8. Placed band as close to natural lashes as possible.					
9. For individual lashes, applied five or six lashes evenly spaced across the lash line, using shorter ones in the inner corner and longer ones toward the outer corner.					
10. Optional: Applied the lower lash bands following the same procedure.					
11. Checked the finished application and made sure client was comfortable with the application.					
12. Completed post-consultation and advised client appropriately for home care.					
Clean-Up and Sanitation					
1. Discarded all disposable supplies and materials.					
2. Disinfected implements.					
3. Cleaned and disinfected brushes.					
4. Placed washable items in the laundry.					
5. Disinfected product containers, used supplies, and workstation.					
6. Washed own hands with soap and warm water.					

19-2

SUPPLIES

- headband
- hand towels
- plastic mixing cup
- distilled water
- small bowl of water
- timer
- brow comb or mascara wand
- eyeliner brush
- disinfectant

PRODUCTS

- cleanser or eye makeup remover
- witch hazel
- petroleum jelly/occlusive cream
- lash tint kits: black for lashes and brown for brows unless client requests otherwise

DISPOSABLES

- cotton swabs (10 to 12)
- round cotton pads (6 to 8)
- paper sheets (1 under each eye)
- baggie

CAUTION!

Do not use tints with aniline derivatives. These are not FDA approved and can cause blindness. Some tints are illegal in the United States, but they may still be available from retailers for use. Do not use them if they are not legal in your region. You may be fined and lose your license. Vegetable dyes are allowed in some regions. Check your local laws to be sure.

Preparation

1 Wash hands.

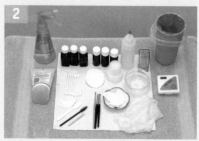

Gather supplies. *(Figure P19-3-1)*

2 Gather and set out supplies (Figure P19-3-1).

3 Wet five cotton pads and five to six cotton swabs. Cut supply amounts in half if doing only one procedure on either the brows or lashes.

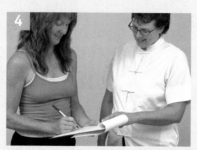

Conduct client consultation. *(Figure P19-3-2)*

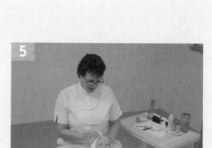

Drape client. *(Figure P19-3-3)*

4 Conduct the client consultation, and have the client sign the release form (Figure P19-3-2).

5 Drape the client with a headband and towel around the neck (Figure P19-3-3).

Procedure

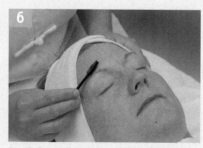

Brush brows in place. *(Figure P19-3-4)*

6 Cleanse the brow and/or lash area. All makeup must be removed and the area clean and dry before applying tint. Brush brows into place (Figure P19-3-4).

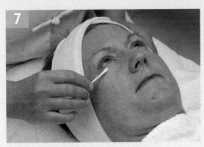

Apply protective cream around area. *(Figure P19–3-5)*

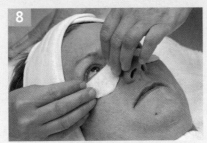

Apply pads. *(Figure P19–3-6)*

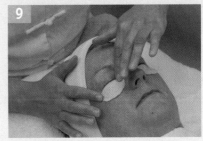

Adjust the pads. *(Figure P19–3-7)*

7 Apply protective cream with a cotton swab directly next to the area where you are tinting to protect the skin, covering the area where you do not want the tint. Do not touch the hairs with cream because this interferes with the color. Apply cream around the brow area. Apply under the eyelashes on the skin below the eye and above the lashes just next to the lash line (Figure P19–3-5).

8 *For lash tinting:* Apply pads under the eyes and over the cream to keep tint from bleeding onto the skin. Use the paper sheaths in the tint kit, or you can make thin cotton pads from cotton rounds. Wet the pads and squeeze out excess water, tearing them so they are half as thick. Then fold in half to make half-moon-shaped pads. You may have to cut or adjust pad shapes to fit under the eyes. Pads should be under the lashes as close to the eye as possible without hiding or interfering with the lower lashes (Figure P19–3-6).

9 Have the client close her eyes, and adjust the pad so it sits next to the eye—not bunched up too close to the eye (Figure P19-3-7). If the pad is too close or too wet, tint may wick into the eye.

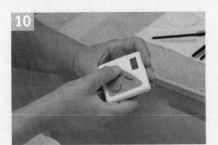

Set timer. *(Figure P19–3-8)*

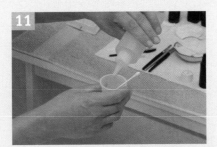

Optional for brows: Dilute tint with water. *(Figure P19–3-9)*

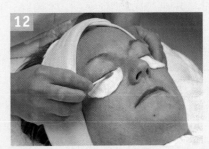

Apply tint. *(Figure P19–3-10)*

10 Set timer according to manufacturer's directions, and have wet pads and cotton swabs ready to use for rinsing (Figure P19–3-8).

11 For brows, the tint can be diluted with water in a 1:1 ratio in a mixing cup to lighten the color (Figure P19–3-9).

12 *Apply tint:* Dip cotton swab or brush applicator into tint (bottle 1), blot excess, apply and carefully saturate the area (Figure P19-3-10).

13 Leave on for three minutes or as directed. Some tint kits have only one bottle and combine the tint and developer into one application. Alter the procedure accordingly. Do not double-dip—use a new applicator each time.

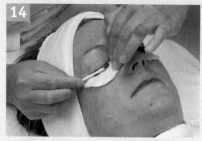

Apply developer. *(Figure P19–3-11)*

14 With a new applicator, apply the developer (bottle 2) for one minute (Figure 19–3-11).

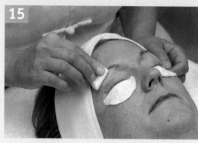

Rinse well. *(Figure P19–3-12)*

15 Rinse each area with water at least three times with wet cotton swabs and cotton pads without dripping into eyes (Figure 19–3-12). *Tip:* Before rinsing, you can replace the under-eye shields if necessary (if color is bleeding through to skin).

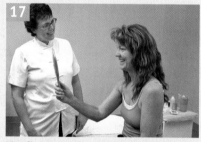

The finished look. *(Figure P19–3-13)*

16 Ask the client if her eyes feel all right, and have her flush them with water at the sink if necessary. It is common for the eyes to feel a little grainy after tinting, so rinsing is a good idea.

17 Show the application to the client. (Figure P19–3-13).

Clean-Up and Sanitation

After the service is completed (and before the clean-up), fill out the client chart, and make retail product suggestions and sales.

18 Wash your hands.

19 Discard all disposable items.

20 Disinfect implements.

21 Clean and disinfect brushes.

22 Place linens in the laundry.

23 Disinfect product containers, supplies, and the workstation.

CAUTION!

To avoid eye damage, do not let tint or water drip into the client's eyes. Have the client keep her eyes closed the whole time.

PROCEDURE 19–3: LASH AND BROW TINTING PROCEDURE

Rubrics are used in education for organizing and interpreting data gathered from observations of student performance. It is a clearly developed scoring document used to differentiate between levels of development in a specific skill performance or behavior. Rubrics are provided in this supplement for use as either a self-assessment tool to aid the student in behavior development or as an educator assessment tool to determine competence. Space is provided to record steps needed for further growth and improvement.

Rate performance according to the following scale:

1 **Development Opportunity:** There is little or no evidence of competency; Assistance is needed; Performance includes multiple errors.

2 **Fundamental:** There is beginning evidence of competency; Task is completed alone; Performance includes few errors.

3 **Competent:** There is detailed and consistent evidence of competency; Task is completed alone; Performance includes rare errors.

4 **Strength:** There is detailed evidence of highly creative, inventive, mature presence of competency.

Space is provided for comments to assist you in improving your performance and achieving a higher rating.

PERFORMANCE ASSESSED	1	2	3	4	IMPROVEMENT PLAN
Preparation					
1. Gathered equipment, supplies, disposables, and products.					
2. Set up room.					
3. Prepared the bed, equipment, and workstation.					
4. Helped client prepare for the service.					
5. Performed consultation and determined client's needs.					
6. Cleansed own hands.					
7. Seated client in makeup chair.					
8. Had client remove contact lenses, if applicable.					
9. Draped client with headband and towel around neck.					
Procedure					
1. Cleansed brow and/or lash area.					
2. Brushed brows into place.					
3. Applied protective cream with cotton swab directly next to area to be tinted to protect skin.					
4. Did not touch lash or brow hairs with protective cream.					
5. Applied pads under the eyes and over the cream to keep tint from bleeding onto skin.					

PERFORMANCE ASSESSED	1	2	3	4	IMPROVEMENT PLAN
6. Applied tint and developer (if applicable) to eyelashes and brows according to manufacturer's directions.					
7. Set timer.					
8. Had wet pads and cotton swabs ready to use for rinsing.					
9. After correct processing time, thoroughly rinsed tint from lashes.					
10. Asked client how her eyes felt and had her flush at sink if necessary.					
11. Showed the finished look to client.					
Clean-Up and Sanitation					
1. Discarded all disposable supplies and materials.					
2. Disinfected implements.					
3. Cleaned and disinfected brushes.					
4. Placed washable items in the laundry.					
5. Disinfected product containers, used supplies, and workstation.					
6. Washed own hands with soap and warm water.					

MILADY'S
STANDARD
ESTHETICS
ADVANCED

Excerpt from
MILADY'S STANDARD
ESTHETICS ADVANCED
STEP-BY-STEP PROCEDURES

ISBN-10: 1-4390-5911-X
ISBN-13: 978-1-4390-5911-1

Order your copy today!

STEP-BY-STEP
PROCEDURES

Procedures List

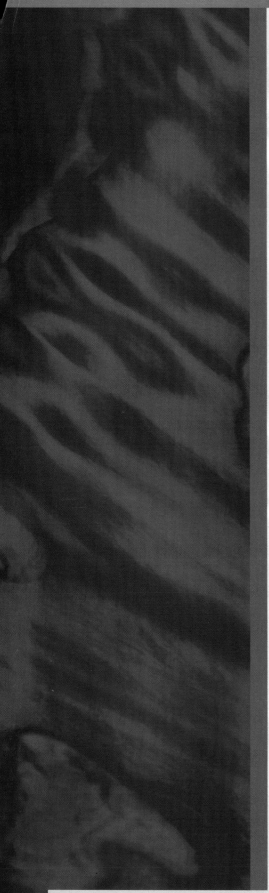

Excerpt from Milady's Standard Esthetics Advanced: Step-by-Step Procedures ISBN-10: 1-4390-5911-X ISBN-13: 978-1-4390-5911. Order your copy today!

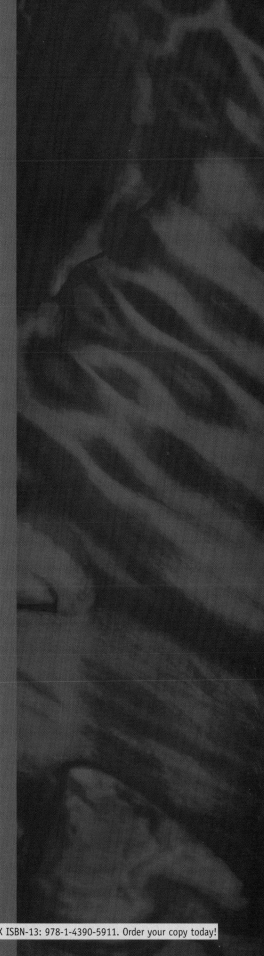

Excerpt from Milady's Standard Esthetics Advanced: Step-by-Step Procedures ISBN-10: 1-4390-5911-X ISBN-13: 978-1-4390-5911. Order your copy today!

This procedure is designed to prepare and soften the impactions for extraction. Thermotherapy facilitates this process and calms the skin following the procedure.

IMPLEMENTS AND MATERIALS

- Cleanser to remove makeup
- Stimulating massage vehicle
- Antiseptic toner
- Typical facial lounge, client draping, and linen setup
- Gloves
- Disposable compresses, cloths, or sponges for removing product
- Water and bowl
- Steamer (optional)
- Treatment brush
- Enzyme exfoliant
- Cotton swabs or comedo extractor
- Serum to facilitate extraction
- Serum to soothe or calm the skin
- Hydrating serum
- Cool globes, high-frequency or sonophoresis
- Hot wet towels
- Cool wet towels
- Sun protection

Preparation

1 Set up the facial lounge with linens.

2 Prepare towels and cotton and gather supplies.

3 Decant and set up products.

Procedure

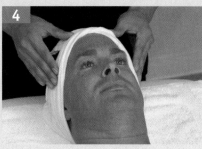

Prepare client.

4 Prepare the client for treatment.

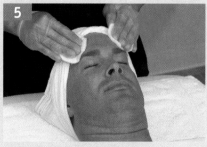

Moisten the skin.

5 Cleanse. Moisten the skin using warm cotton compresses or sponges.

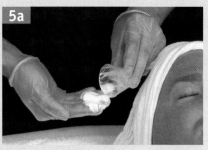

Apply a cleanser.

a. Apply a cleanser suitable to remove makeup with your gloved hands (optional).

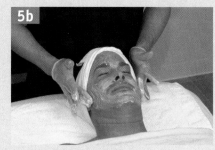

Massage the cleanser.

b. Massage the cleanser to loosen makeup.

Excerpt from Milady's Standard Esthetics Advanced: Step-by-Step Procedures ISBN-10: 1-4390-5911-X ISBN-13: 978-1-4390-5911. Order your copy today!

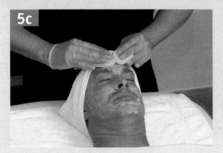

Remove the cleanser.

    c. Remove the cleanser using a warm cloth, sponges, or compresses.

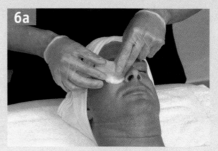

Place eye pads on eyes.

6 Analysis and consultation.

    a. Place moistened eye pads on eyes.

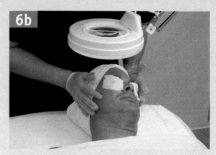

Examine skin.

    b. Examine the client's skin under magnifying lamp. Observe the level of sensitivity and skin response to cleansing. Confirm that the selected products will be appropriate.

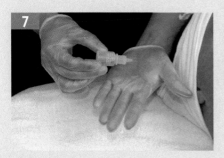

Apply a serum.

7 Apply a serum designed to loosen impactions. If you use warm steam, stand at a distance of 18 to 20 inches from the client's face.

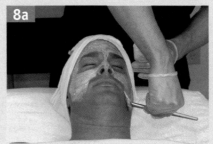

Use an enzyme exfoliant.

8 Exfoliation.

    a. Use an enzyme exfoliant following manufacturer's guidelines.

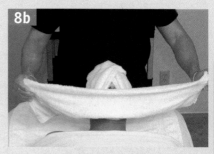

Wrap the face in a classical barber wrap.

    b. Wrap the face in two hot towels in a classical barber wrap. The first towel should be hot but comfortable. Place the second towel on top of the first. It should be as hot as you can handle.

16–1

    c. Leave the towel on the skin for approximately 8 to 10 minutes. If the towel cools too quickly, use steam to keep it warm or replace the top towel with a fresh one.

    d. Remove top towel.

    e. Use the lower towel to remove enzyme from the skin.

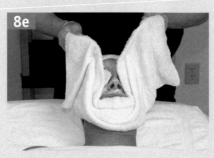

Remove enzyme.

continues on next page

Excerpt from Milady's Standard Esthetics Advanced: Step-by-Step Procedures ISBN-10: 1-4390-5911-X ISBN-13: 978-1-4390-5911. Order your copy today!

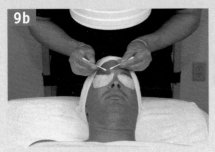

Perform extraction.

9 Extraction. Before starting, refresh gloves if necessary.

   a. Apply a pre-extraction serum if desired. Follow manufacturer's guidelines.

   b. Use cotton swab technique or comedone extractor to perform extraction.

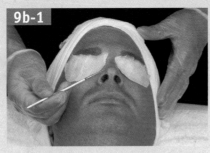

Continue to perform extractions.

   c. If skin begins to welt, redden severely, or swell, stop extraction immediately.

   d. Limit the extraction to 5 to 10 minutes only, particularly during the first visit.

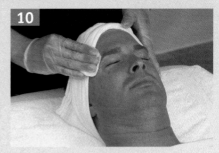

Wipe skin with toner.

10 Wipe the skin with an antiseptic toner.

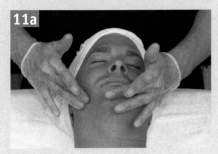

Apply serum.

11 Calm.

   a. Apply soothing serum.

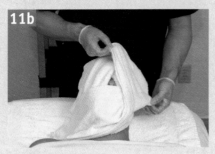

Apply cold wet towels.

   b. Apply cold wet towels wrapping the face in classical barber wrap. As an alternative, you can use cold globes, slowly stroking across the entire face, one area at a time.

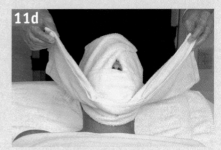

Remove towels.

   c. Allow the skin to calm about 10 minutes.

   d. Remove towels.

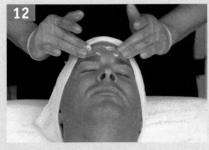

Apply sunscreen.

12 Apply a hydrating fluid and sunscreen.

Post-Procedure

13 Advise the client to treat any extracted area carefully, avoiding touching it to minimize contamination with bacteria.

14 Remind the client to avoid the sun.

15 Determine if the client is using appropriate home-care products for his or her skin.

Clean-Up and Disinfection

16 Follow clean-up and disinfection procedures in accordance with state guidelines.

17 Reset and prepare the room for the next client.

Excerpt from Milady's Standard Esthetics Advanced: Step-by-Step Procedures ISBN-10: 1-4390-5911-X ISBN-13: 978-1-4390-5911. Order your copy today!